SLIM SUPPLE & STRONG

YOUR COMPLETE STEP BY STEP GUIDE
TO THE **NEW YOU**

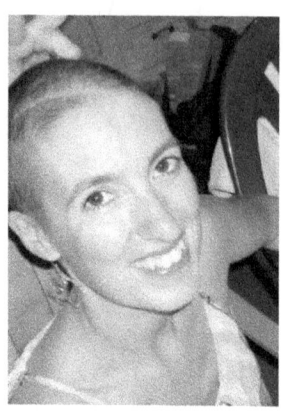

It came as quite a surprise to get the phone call that announced my breast cancer. At the age of 33, with no family history and having breastfed all three of my daughters, It was unimaginable to get the big ' C ' diagnosis. I was otherwise physically fit and healthy. Then the fight for my life began and today I am still undergoing treatment. The prognosis is excellent and I attribute my success and sanity to my physical and emotional health. I believe that It was my good physical condition that helped to speed up my recovery and reduce the severity of symptoms produced from the treatments for my breast cancer. It helped me cope physically and mentally with the months of chemotherapy, surgery and radiotherapy. Walking and swimming helped with the nausea and fatigue from chemotherapy. After surgery, exercises helped retain the range of motion (mobility) in my limbs. During radiotherapy walking increased both my energy and self esteem during the final stages of treatment. Exercise releases serotonin, which makes you happy and It also boosts your immune system, all excellent reasons for investing in your body's health, so that we are better equipped to cope with whatever life throws at us. After over 11 months of hospital visits, stays and treatments I am thoroughly enjoying a variety of exercise and I am seeing my energy return and starting to trust my body again. Conditioning work with bands, cycling, zumba, walking and resistance training are all part of the fun, It puts a smile on my face to think about It.

Many years ago I had the pleasure of working and training with a very dedicated and passionate man. During the time we worked together he decided that there was a great need for producing a book to help simplify and clarify how to improve physical health and wellbeing. I am proud to be part of this book.

Samantha Slade

Personal Trainer & Group Exercise Instructor

Breast Cancer Survivor & Mother of 3

SLIM SUPPLE & STRONG

YOUR COMPLETE STEP BY STEP GUIDE TO THE *NEW YOU*

Gary Richards

FORWARD

As a fitness professional I have become increasingly astounded as to the number of publications that are continually hitting the market professing to have the answer to weight loss, well-being and general fitness. Low carbohydrate diets are sweeping the world, while the great percentage of people who require help will only become sicker and more disillusioned as their body's primary source of fuel (carbohydrate) is withheld. Our kids are coming through with massive obesity problems and growing up with this rubbish. What hope have they got as they are fed with fad after fad, which are after all, usually only private money making episodes. Carbohydrate in itself is not fattening and supplies 16 Kilojoules per gram of energy, where as fat supplies Kilojoules at a rate of 37 per gram. It is the overall Calorie (Kilojoule) energy input that we are interested in. A lack of carbohydrate can cause a multitude of problems such as Kidney damage, Bone weakness, Bad breath, Diarrhoea and dizzy spells just to name a few. Without the Vitamins, Minerals and Fibre that carbohydrates supply to our bodies serious problems are going to set in at some point, particularly as the majority of health professionals are aware, most of our problems stem from one deficiency or another or a combination of them. Worse still the body deprived of it's primary source of energy can begin to look for energy by breaking down your lean muscle mass for fuel. Now because the low-Carb diet is not sustainable you ultimately give it up and your lean muscle mass is not recovered and the *subsequent weight gain will be all fat.* That's how you end up fatter than you were before you started the fad diet.

The takeaway food industry has had a lot to answer for, as has the dairy industry over the years, although much improved in recent times. Fat has flavour, so what happens when they are forced to regulate the amount of saturated fat? In goes the sugar, and what happens when we get bombarded with processed sugar? Bring on the Diabetes, the poor old pancreas must be the busiest organ of all as it continually secretes insulin to lower blood sugar levels. Governments are going to have to be forced by their appropriate electorates to address these huge problems of which weigh heavily on contemporary society as we know it. As a great percentage of our kids are getting sick at such a vulnerable age, society in future is not going to be able to handle such a massive sickness industry. Health problems backed up by our latest science must be heavily promoted by Governments at all levels to combat this tirade of mis-information.

Now on a happier note, Slim Supple & Strong is a wholistic publication in the sense that it addresses the balances that are required for a person to actually be what they want to be. Through good science such as the Glycaemic Index, thoroughly researched food values and professional exercise programs, Slim, Supple & Strong is put together in such a way that it flows and gives the reader a true sense of clarity and direction. Most people are very busy in today's society, they havn't the time to work out how many calories in this meal, how many grams of protein or carbohydrate is in this one, or how do these foods rate on the glycaemic index. Slim Supple & Strong is designed to ensure continuity and sustainability of the new lifestyle the reader has embarked apon.

This edition is dedicated to getting the participant to a point where they have obtained their new weight, mastered simple resistance exercises, learn't correct stretching techniques, performed basic yoga and pilates positions and obtained some cardiovascular fitness. At this stage the participant is eating to keep up their calorie count to match what their body requires, basically keeping things on an even keel, i.e energy in and energy out being equal. At this stage your body is really toning up and you are feeling new levels of self esteem and a deep inner confidence. If you so wish, you can specialise in your area of choice as your lean muscle mass has increased, your aerobic capability has vastly improved, bone density has increased and you have obtained a firm toned body with stronger ligaments and joints, thus completing the *new sustainable forever you.*

I'm not going to bore you with figures but let's not kid ourselves, over half of our total population are seriously overweight or obese. We've just recently won the premiership, yes we are now officially the fattest country in the world. A huge percentage of our kids are staring the big 4 right in the eye.

- HEART DISEASE
- DIABETES
- HIGH BLOOD PRESSURE
- CHOLESTEROL

You know as well as I do that it all comes down to your eating plan and lifestyle. Only a small percentage are unlucky enough to suffer from a predominantly genetical condition affecting their metabolism. We all know the reasons why, with this modern age of technology, takeaway foods, processed foods, the list goes on and on. I know all the excuses, as a fitness trainer I've heard the lot, but in saying that I also appreciate the stresses placed on people in this modern era, however if you have the desire to live long, happy, healthy and rewarding life you must :

BECOME SLIM SUPPLE & STRONG

The beauty of this straightforward, scientifically based book is in it's simplicity and balance. Follow it to the letter and you will notice the excess fat begin to fall off you and your energy levels begin to rise.

- You begin to feel better about yourself
- You start to tone up as the exercises kick in
- The world begins to look a little brighter
- Not as many people seem to annoy you anymore
- You begin to develop a deep inner confidence
- Most of all it is totally sustainable

Once you have finished this book and created new patterns in your life, it is not only sustainable but irreversible, the **NEW YOU** is taking shape without fad diets, without guilt trips, without society pressures and anxiety becomes a distant mirage.

ACKNOWLEDGEMENTS

I would like to thank Sandra Lang and Samantha Slade for their time and expertise in performing the exercise demonstrations during the photo shoot at Palm Cove North Queensland Australia. Also a special thanks to my partner Ai Takezawa for her many hours of imput and layout on the computer.

Since that photo shoot, Samantha was diagnosed with breast cancer and has not only survived but is now back working as a personal trainer and group exercise instructor whilst still under treatment. She is an inspiration to all she comes into contact with and a great ambassador for the cause.

Best Regards to all

Gary Richards

Author

Contents

DIET FACTS

- All fad diets are unsustainable
- Prolonged exposure to no carbohydrate diets will cause Bad breath, Kidney damage, Bone weakness, Diarrhoea and dizzy spells
- Your body, deprived of it's principal energy source (carbohydrates) will look for energy by breaking down protein (your own lean muscle mass)
- On coming off a no carbohydrate diet, muscle atrophy (loss) will not be recovered as water weight loss is quickly replaced and the subsequent weight gain will be ' Fat '
- Any diet will rarely be effective if the person is left in a constant state of Feeling hungry
- If a diet is too complicated people will not adhere to it
- Fat is actually an important pre-requisite for the digestive process, it is the amount and the type that we must control
- Consume only monounsaturated, polyunsaturated fats and the omega 3's
- Carbohydrates are converted by your body into it's primary energy source, Glucose, and are rich in Fibre, Minerals, Vitamins and Antioxidants
- Processed foods are digested by the body quickly and hunger returns soon after consumption. Look for foods high in both soluble and insoluble fibre
- We must all learn to recognise Slow release foods that break down at a steady rate in the digestive system. Thus we have the :

'GLYCAEMIC INDEX'

THE GLYCAEMIC INDEX

The speed at which food is digested and broken down into glucose is given an index 1 – 100. Sugar is set at 100 and all other foods are measured against it. The body quickly converts high G.I foods into glucose which is when the pancreas releases insulin. Insulin firstly diverts glucose to body tissues for immediate use, then stores the remainder as FAT.

- Insulin secondly prevents the conversion of body fat back into glucose.
- Therefore to lose weight you must keep insulin levels low.
- To keep insulin levels low you must stay with Low G.I foods of which break down at a slow even rate so that sudden high levels of glucose are not converted to Fat. Conversion of fat into energy is assisted therefore in a low insulin environment.
- The key to successful weight loss through diet is the combination of low G.I and Low Calorie foods.
- A balanced diet contains components that act as a brake in the digestive process of a food, an example being the amount of fibre which contributes to a Low G.I rating.
- Protein and fat also act as a brake in the digestive process, however we must be careful as fat contains many more calories than proteins and carbohydrates.
- The other consideration is the Type of fat.

Protein should be included with all meals, examples being lean low fat meats, low fat yoghurt, tofu, soy and whey protein powder, low fat cottage cheese and omega 3 eggs. Preferably protein should be sourced from both animal and vegetable products, being soy and whey respectively.

GENERAL INFORMATION

The following is general information for you to keep in mind as you follow your path to success. You do not want to interrupt your diet and exercise routines later on through constantly searching for basic information. Remember that Simplicity and Clarity is what we are all about.

Always have 3 meals a day

- Always use a substitute for sugar
- Only drink water, low calorie drinks and skimmed milk in stage 1.
- Generally try to drink 1.5 – 2.0 litres / day of water
- Good hydration means more calories burnt
- Don't waste your calorie allocation on drinks, they do not satisfy hunger.
- No alcohol in stage 1, it is full of empty calories.
- Serving size for meat is 100g or roughly the size of the palm of your hand.
- Serving size for pasta and rice 50g (dry)
- One calorie = 4.2 Kilojoules of energy.
- Carbohydrates are not fattening, excess Cal/Kilojoules are fattening.
- Only 4 vegetables have a high G.I, parsnips, Swedes, pumpkin & turnip.
- Plain dark chocolate has a low G.I, eat sparingly it is high in fat.
- Try green tea as recent science says that caffeine can increase insulin.
- Every gram of fibre digested burns 29 Kilojoules of energy.
- Make sure you have some protein with every meal.
- Eat only quality breads, granary, barley, rye, soya and wheat tortilla wraps.
- Portions: Vegetables 50%, Meat 25%, Pasta, Rice, Potatoes 25%

Finally, if you must have a high G.I food, have something acidic with it such as grapefruit.

MOTIVATION GOALS RESULTS

This is what we are about, keeping up our motivation and attaining our goals. Keeping track of our progress is an important and motivating habit that we are going to adopt.

All you require is a standard, material type tape measure and a set of reliable scales. On the following page is a record sheet for you to photocopy. To keep to our original pledge of simplicity only your weight and waist measurement will be required. Always measure in the same place (eg navel or just above) and weigh at the same time (eg first thing in the morning before breakfast)

On the next page is another record sheet for you to keep track of your eating patterns on a daily basis. Later on you will use another sheet to record your weekly exercise routine, so at a glance you will able to see the new you taking shape. I will get into the exercise prescription for you a little later, our priority at this stage is to get you to your correct weight with the assistance of an easy and pleasurable exercise routine. I would like add here that your new eating plan will give you unbelievable extra energy and this in turn makes the exercise much easier to perform. Not far down the track you will look forward to your exercise with a new zest.

As you have probably already gathered we are being totally realistic here. As stated in the diet facts earlier fad diets are not sustainable, and as you have more than likely experienced yourself, once stopping the diet you end up fatter than you were before. Now we are not all goody goody's and you will more than likely break out every now and then, but do not let it get to you, remind yourself that after this first stage things become more liberal. Get back on board and stay with the 90-10 rule minimum, so you have played up 10% of the time, don't send yourself down a self destructive, guilt ridden path of anxiety.

OK, LET'S GET OUR SHOPPING LIST TOGETHER

MEASUREMENT CHART

DATE	WEEK No.	WEIGHT	WAIST	COMMENTS
	1			
	2			
	3			
	4			
	5			
	6			
	7			
	8			
	9			
	10			
	11			
	12			
	13			
	14			
	15			
	16			
	17			
	18			
	19			
	20			

FOOD CHART

WEEK No.

NAME:

DAY	DATE	BREAKFAST	SNACK	LUNCH	SNACK	DINNER	SNACK
MONDAY							
NOTES							
TUESDAY							
NOTES							
WEDNESDAY							
NOTES							
THURSDAY							
NOTES							
FRIDAY							
NOTES							
SATURDAY							
NOTES							
SUNDAY							
NOTES							

ALLOWABLE FOODS LIST

All Bran
Apple & Bran Muffins
Apples
Almonds (limited)
All Spices (used sparingly)
Apple Sauce (unsweetened)
Asparagus
Aubergine
Alfalfa
Bread (100% stoneground or a quality whole grain)
Basmati Rice
Beans (fresh & most canned beans, low fat, drained & rinsed)
Baking Powder & Soda
Blueberries & Blackberries (not canned in syrup)
Black Pepper Corns
Bottled Water
Buttermilk
Broccoli
Brussel Sprouts
Buckwheat Flour
Buckwheat
Bacon (lean back rashers)
Cabbage
Carrots
Cauliflour
Celery
Cherries
Cherrie Tomatoes
Cheese (fat free)
Chicken Breast (skinless)
Cottage Cheese (fat free)
Chilles
Courgettes
Cucumber
Cocoa
Coffee (de-caffeinated)
Cold pressed olive oil (extra virgin)
Carob

Canola spread (light) and use sparingly
Extra Extra Lean Mince
Fettuccine Pasta
Flavoured Vinegars
Frozen Yoghurt (fat & sugar free)
Fromage Frais
Filtered Water
Grapefruit
Grapes (white)
Green Tea
Ham (lean deli)
Hazelnuts
Ice-Cream (fat & sugar free)
Larissa Paste
Lean Beef & Ham
Leeks
Limes
Lemons
Lettuce
Mandarins
Margarine (non-hydrogenated) Light
Mayonaise (fat free)
Mushrooms
New Potatoes only (boiled)
Non-Fat yoghurt (preferably sugar-free)
Oat Bran
Olives
Olive Oil (extra virgin, preferably cold pressed used sparingly)
Old Style Oats
Onions
Omega 3 Eggs (no more than 5 whole eggs per week)
Oranges
Parmesan Cheese (very sparingly)
Pasta (fetticine, spag, penne, maca, vermicelli, linguine) limited & wholemeal
Peaches
Peas
Pearl Barley
Peppers
Plums
Porridge (old style oats)

Protein Powder (soy or whey)
Potatoes (new, boiled)
Pickles
Raspberries
Rapeseed Oil
Raisins (only a few for cooking e.g muffins)
Raw Vegetables
Red Onions
Rice (Brown, Longrain, Wild)
Salad Dressings (fat-free) or vinegar & olive oil
Seafood (no additives or batters) See List for Stage 1
Sea Salt
Skimmed Milk
Sliced Almonds
Soy Beans
Soy Milk (low-fat)
Soy Protein Powder
Soda Water
Soft Drinks (diet only) moderation
Soups (chunky bean, vegetable and pasta)
Spices & Herbs
Spinach
Sugar Snap Peas
Sweet Potato
Teas (all teas)
Tomatoes
Tofu
Turkey Breast (skinless)
Vegetables (all vegetables except pumpkin, Swedes, large potatoes and parsnips)
Veal (lean cuts)
Vegetarian Chilli
Vegetable Sprays
Whole Wheat Breadcrumbs
Wheat Tortilla wrap
Whole Meal Flour
Wheat Bran
Zuchini

SEAFOOD SHOPPING LIST

I have decided to add this seafood shopping list for you. It is an added bonus if you are a seafood fan as the general health and nutritional benefits of seafood are well documented. Please remember, NO coatings or deep frying.

As carbohydrates and fibre are minimal and of little consequence with seafood, the following list has been carefully compiled and are the lowest in fat and calorie content. These are the most suitable for the early stages , later on I will introduce other products for you, such as good oily mackerel, but 100g of smoked mackerel for example contains 31g Fat and1465 Kj, as against 100g of Cod which contains 1g of fat and only 420Kg.

Anchovies (in brine)

Blue Grenadier

Cod (baked or grilled)

Caviar (black in brine)

Crab (fresh or canned)

Flounder (baked or grilled)

Leatherjacket (steamed or poached)

Ling (steamed or poached)

Lobster

Mussels (steamed or boiled)

Ocean Perch (baked or grilled)

Oysters (raw)

Octopus (steamed)

Prawns (school prawns only)

Pike (grilled)

Scallops (steamed or boiled)

Scampi (steamed, boiled or grilled)

Snapper (grilled or baked)

Trout (rainbow, grilled or baked)

Tuna (canned in brine)

Whiting (baked or grilled

CUPBOARD CLEANING

I would like you to clean out your food cupboards prior to going shopping armed with your new eat only list. If you are in a family situation and they are not involved with your new program, allocate a separate cupboard for yourself and stock only the allowable foods.

A SHOPPING YOU WILL GO

You do not have to buy everything on the list immediately, grab the essentials like skim milk, all bran or oats, fruits, vegetables, lean meats, bread and salads.

From the recipes and your own imagination work out what meals you are going to prepare for the first few days and buy accordingly. Have fun and experiment. If you are interested in a food that you are unfamiliar with or you want try something that is not on the list make sure that it is :

A / Low fat (especially saturated fat)
B / Low calorie
C / High fibre

Re calorie content per serving, make sure the serving size is a reasonable one.

I have spent many hours researching the foods on your list and they are there only because they have met strict criteria, so please do not try to re-invent the wheel as they say. The criteria for including a food is not just that it has a low G.I, it must be within certain limits in regard to fat (both saturated & unsaturated) fibre content, calories and nutritional value.

A great example of this is good old peanut butter, sure a low G.I but it is very calorie dense and not suitable in the early stages, however ok for kids on the go. Alcohol and sugar are high energy and high calorie foods, but are what we call empty calories as the energy units are lacking in vitamins and minerals.

SO GRAB THAT TROLLEY AND LET'S ROLL

BREAKFAST

PORRIDGE (1 SERVE)

50g (1 ¾ oz) rolled oats (the real big flaked oats)

Follow directions on packet.

Use only water & skimmed milk.

To make it a bit more interesting try mixing in fat free yoghurt, 1 tbsp sliced almonds, fresh fruit pieces, or your allowable berries.

This is the breakfast you really should be aiming for as often as possible, it will follow you around all morning.

A grapefruit or whole orange instead of juice, as this provides more fibre and less calories, finished off with your favourite cup of tea with skimmed milk and sugar substitute if required, (a great anti-oxidant)

MUESLI

Soak your oats in skimmed milk overnight, then mix in the fruit, berries, sliced almonds and sweetener (preferably aspartame)

50g (13/4 oz) rolled oats
180ml (6 fl oz) skimmed milk
125g (4 oz) diced pear, apples or berries
1 tbsp sliced almonds
180g (6 oz) fat free yoghurt

These two make a wonderfully nourishing breakfast and get you off to great start.

OMELETTE (1 SERVE)

The following is your basic omelette recipe. Omega 3 eggs are a wonderful food to use, if you can't find them use 1 whole egg with two egg whites.

This is a very versatile breakfast as any of your foods on the list can be added. You can come up with a Mexicana, an Italiano or a Vegetarian. Use the same mixture for your scrambled eggs (mix in the pan instead)

2 tsp olive oil

3 eggs

60 m (2 fl oz) skimmed milk

Using this recipe as a base you may add your favourite vegetables, bacon (back) lean ham, turkey or chicken breast.

Other ingredients could be tomato puree, red and green peppers, chillies or chilli powder, canned beans or sliced mushrooms. If adding chedder or mozzarella cheese use no more than 30g (10oz)

Saute your vegetables and keep aside, pour in mixture then add ingredients as omelette starts to firm.

Top off your breakfast with some fresh fruit, a glass of skimmed milk or fat-free yoghurt followed by de-caffienated coffee or tea (green tea is a great anti-oxidant and assists in burning calories)

I'M OUT OF HERE

At least take the time to grab some low-fat fruit yoghurt and some fresh fruit.

OR

A sachet (40g) of instant porridge with skim milk and a piece of fruit.

HIGH FIBRE COLD CEREAL

80g (2 ½ oz) All Bran

180 ml (6 fl oz) skimmed milk

120g (4 oz) fresh fruit pieces, pears, peaches, strawberries, blueberries.

1 tbsp sliced almonds and sweetener (e.g aspartame) if required.

Compliment this breakfast with a serve of fat free yoghurt or alternatively add to your cereal.

You could finish off with a slice of toast (wholemeal) with a light spread of canola and reduced fat and sugar free fruit jam, with your favourite hot drink, decaffeinated coffee or tea.

SUNDAY SPECIAL COOKED BREAKFAST

2 Eggs scrambled, poached or boiled (try for omega 3 eggs)

Grilled or sautéed mushrooms

Grilled tomato

1 rasher of lean back bacon

1 slice of toast (wholegrain / wholemeal) light canola spread

Piece of fruit with decaffeinated coffee.

LUNCH

Always include some protein with your salads and vegetables like chicken or turkey breast (skinless) lean ham, fish (no coatings) low fat cottage cheese or beans.

Stay strictly with your wholegrain / wholemeal breads, canola light spreads, and low fat / light salad dressings. If unavailable use olive oil and red wine vinegar.

Chunky vegetable soups together with a salad makes an ideal lunch.

Tuna (canned in brine) and salad sandwich, wholegrain bread with canola light.

Include a piece of fresh fruit or tub of non-fat yoghurt with a glass of skimmed milk or water.

CRAB AND SALAD TORTILLA WRAP

Wheat or wholemeal tortilla wrap spread with canola light.

50g (2 oz) fresh or canned crab meat

Favourite salad mix.

Serve with canned mixed beans or red kidney beans (drained & rinsed) you can add a bit of get up and go with chilli powder, garlic, olive oil and lemon.

SASSY TOMATO AND LENTIL SOUP

210g (7oz) can of diced tomatoes / 240g (8oz) red lentils / 1 lge red onion / 1 chopped clove of garlic / 1 tbsp olive oil / 1 stick celery / chilli to taste / ground cumin / paprika / salt & pepper / garnished with chopped coriander.

Soak lentils in bowl of water while you are sautéing the celery, garlic and onion in the olive oil. Add drained lentils to the vegetable pan with the chopped tomatoes mix and add the remaining spices. Cover and simmer until lentils are soft (approx 30 min)

CHICKEN CAESAR SALAD

120g (4 oz) skinless chicken breast (grilled)

Plenty lettuce

Cherry Tomatoes

No more than 15g (½ oz) parmesan cheese

1 tbsn low-fat Caesar salad dressing

Top off with a container of healthy soup (your tomato & lentil soup)

THAI BEEF SALAD

100g of lean beef

Green onions, bean sprouts, cherry tomatoes, cucumber, mint and coriander leaves.

Slice beef into thin strips and quickly fry in 1 tbsp olive oil and combine.

ASIAN STIR – FRY

100g skinless turkey or chicken breast cubed.

1 tblsp olive oil

Carrots / cauliflour / broccoli / mushrooms / onions / chillies

Or mixed frozen vegetables approx 300g (10 oz)

Stir fry vegetables adding yellow, red and green peppers for flavour and colour.

Add grated root ginger and a touch of soy sauce with salt and pepper.

Add the chicken or turkey and simmer until cooked.

DINNER

Unless stated otherwise recipes are for one person. The preferred choice of meats are skinless chicken and turkey breast with a small amount of lean steak. You will notice quite a lot of fish and seafood dishes.

Please remember your ratios :

Vegetables 50%

Potatoes / Pasta / Rice 25%

Poultry / Meat / Fish 25%

BARBEQUED STEAK

120g / 4oz lean steak, totally trimmed of fat

3 small boiled new potatoes

Onions / field mushrooms / asparagus / brussel sprouts / green beans and broccoli

While your new potatoes are boiling, steam, boil or microwave the brussel sprouts, beans, broccoli and fresh asparagus.

In a non-stick pan sauté the onions and mushrooms in a small amount of water. These three jobs could be handled by your willing assistant whilst you are barbequing the steaks. A good tip is to finish off your steaks on the grilling section allowing any fat to drain prior to serving.

OR

While the barbie is warming up have a pan of chipped sweet potatoes dry roasting in the oven, throw on your sirloin and serve with your favourite salad and or vegetables.

As I said earlier please stay with beef as pork and lamb tend to have a higher fat content, and even then keep it down and only buy the extra, extra lean mince.

Also remember not to make the fatal mistake of allowing the pasta or rice to dominate the dish thereby ruining your ratios.

GRILLED CHICKEN BREAST WITH PEARL BARLEY BASE (SERVES 2)

2 Skinless chicken breasts

60g (2 oz) pearl barley cooked

1 tbls olive oil

Chilli to taste (powder or chopped whole chilli)

1 red onion chopped

2 tbls chopped coriander

1 red pepper

Juice of one lime with the rind grated

Have the barley cooking as per instructions on packet

Brush chicken lightly with olive oil, then grill until golden brown

Stir oil / chopped red onion / chilli / coriander / red pepper and lime juice with grated rind into the barley.

Serve barley with sliced chicken breast and garnish with chopped parsley.

MINESTRONE WITH MEATBALLS (SERVES 4)

400g lean lean lean beef mince

2 celery sticks chopped

1 green capsicum chopped and fresh basil

1 large carrot chopped

Two 400g cans crushed tomatoes

1 large red onion chopped and 2 cloves of garlic crushed.

Combine half the onions and half the garlic with the mince and make into small meat balls. In a lightly oiled non-stick pan cook until nice and brown, remove from pan.

Cook remaining garlic, onion, carrot, capsicum and celery in pan until tender then add tomatoes and bring to the boil.

Return meatballs to pan, reduce heat, simmer uncovered until cooked then stir in chopped basil.

POACHED COD IN PARSLEY SAUCE

100g (4oz) cod steak

1 tbls chopped parsley

50g (2oz) buckwheat

Broccoli / carrots / cauliflower

3 tbls white wine

1 tbls light canola spread

Melt the canola and add white wine in non-stick pan
Poach cod steak in pan with chopped parsley
Serve with buckwheat and vegetables.

STEAMED COD WITH TOMATOES AND LENTILS

100g (4 oz) cod steak

100g (4 oz) green lentils (canned / drained)

8 cherry tomatoes

50g (2 oz) mushrooms

50g (2 oz) leek (sliced into strips)

25g (1 oz) celery (chopped finely)

½ clove garlic (chopped finely)

1 tbls olive oil

½ red onion (chopped finely)

1 tsp fresh parsley

1 tsp thyme

Any firm white flesh fish off your list may be used for this recipe.

Start steaming the cod steak (approx 15 min) Heat olive oil in a frypan and cook onion until soft, adding the garlic, celery and leek, cooking for a couple of minutes. Add sliced mushrooms, a bit of water as necessary and cook for a further 3 minutes.

Finally add lentils, thyme, parsley and tomatoes and cook for a further 3 minutes. Pour mixture onto plate placing cod on top and season to taste.

STEAMED TROUT WITH CORIANDER AND GINGER

2 whole rainbow trout (approx 360g / 12 oz each) cleaned

Piece of ginger (approx 5cm or 2 inches long) cut into matchsticks

2 limes cut into thin slices

30g or 1oz sugar replacement (eg aspartame)

60ml / 2 fl oz lime juice (about ¼ cup) plus the rind of 1 lime cut into strips

10g or ¼ oz (approx 1/3 cup) fresh coriander leaves

Preheat oven to 180 C (350 F)

With the lime slices and some of the ginger fill the fish cavity

Wrap the fish in foil and bake approx 30 min

Mix the lime juice and sugar substitute with 250ml (8fl oz) water in a small pan until dissolved, then bring to the boil, reducing heat and simmering until syrupy (approx 10 min)

Stir in the remaining lime strips and ginger

Place fish on plate covering with fresh coriander leaves and pour over syrup

Serve with capsicum, snow peas and fresh asparagus or your favourite salad or as a side dish.

SWEET POTATO AND SPINACH BAKE

250g / 10oz sweet potato, peeled and cut in half

200g / 8oz fresh spinach

1 whole nutmeg

60g / 2oz low-fat fromage frais

Preheat oven to 180 C / 350 F while partly boiling the sweet potato, allow to cool and cut into thin slices.

Place the spinach into boiling water (30 sec only, just enough to wilt it) and drain

In an oven proof dish place a third of the spinach at the bottom, grating a little nutmeg over it, then spread 1/3 of the fromage on top. Add 1/3 of the sweet potato slices as a layer, repeat layers and bake 35 – 40 minutes

BEEF AND VEGETABLE CASSEROLE (SERVES 6)

500g (1 lb) lean round steak

500g (1 lb) sweet potatoes

1 onion sliced, 3 cloves of garlic

440g (14 oz) can chopped tomatoes

240g (8oz) mushrooms (lge pieces)

240g (8 oz) yellow squash (chunky pieces)

4 zucchini (chunky pieces)

3 lge carrots

2 teaspoons ground cumin

2 bay leaves

1 teaspoon dried thyme

3 tbls tomato paste

½ cup (130 ml red wine)

½ cup (20g) chopped parsley

Preheat oven to 180 C / 350 F, cut steak into 2cm (¾ inch) cubes after removing any fat and sinew. Spray your non-stick frypan with cooking oil and in small lots, brown all the meat pieces then set aside.

Give the pan another light spray and cook the onion until just golden, adding next the garlic, cumin, bay leaves and thyme, stir for 2 minutes.

Now return the meat together with any juices to pan making sure all pieces are well coated with the spices.

Add 375ml / 12fl oz of water together with the can of chopped tomato, stirring until thickened (about 10 mins)

Mix with tomato paste, wine and all vegetables in a large casserole dish. Cover and bake for 1 hour then take out of oven, give it a good stir and bake for a further 20 minutes uncovered.

Finally remove the bay leaves and stir in the parsley before serving.

This is a very wholesome dish which can be heated up for further meals, can be eaten for lunch or dinner and contains protein, carbohydrate and fibre.

HOW MUCH SHOULD I LOSE ?

Most health professionals use the BMI (Body Mass Index) as a guide to a person's ideal weight. This method is surprisingly accurate, particularly when compared to the old height by weight guide which is just not accurate enough.

Your BMI can be easily calculated using the following equation.

Weight (Kg) divided by Height (m squared) = BMI

Eg : 78 Kg divided by 1.75m times 1.75 = 26 BMI

BMI   Below 18   Underweight

      18 - 24   Ideal Weight Range

      25 - 29   Overweight

      30 - 40   Obese

      Over 40   Excessively Obese

The calculation of your weight range via the BMI index is quite accurate for most people, however there are exceptions.

For example an unusually short person who is heavily muscled would give an incorrect reading as the scale is interpreting lean muscle mass as body fat. And as with older people, degeneration of muscle mass and tissues is normal but it could give a reading as underweight even though that person is quite healthy.

Interestingly, the above example is myself and I know that I am about 5 kg over weight and if this was lost (which it will be) would bring me into the ideal weight range.

To find your ideal weight, refer to the table on the following page. Firstly find your height at top of page, then run your finger down the column and stop at your weight. The figure you now have is your BMI.

Refer this to the table (I know you probably won't be happy) now run your finger back up the column until you are within the 18 – 24 range, then across to that weight.

The difference between the two weights is ideally what you should lose.

WEIGHT HEIGHT- FEET & INCHES / CENTEMETRES

St lb's	Kilo's	4'8"	4'10"	5'0"	5'2"	5'3"	5'4"	5'5"	5'6"	5'7"	5'8"	5'9"	5'10"	5'11"	6'0"	6'2"	6'4"
		142	147	152	157	160	163	165	168	170	173	175	178	180	183	188	193
7.3	46	22	21	19	18	17	17	16	16	15	15	14	14	14	13	13	12
7.7	48	23	21	20	19	18	18	17	16	16	16	15	15	14	14	13	12
7.10	49	24	22	21	19	19	18	18	17	16	16	15	15	15	14	13	13
8.0	51	25	23	21	20	19	19	18	18	17	17	16	16	15	15	14	13
8.3	52	25	24	22	21	20	19	19	18	18	17	17	16	16	15	14	14
8.7	54	26	24	23	21	21	20	19	19	18	18	17	17	16	16	15	14
8.10	55	27	25	23	22	21	20	20	19	19	18	18	17	17	16	15	14
9.3	59	28	27	25	23	22	22	21	20	20	19	19	18	18	17	16	15
9.7	60	29	27	26	24	23	22	22	21	20	20	19	19	18	18	17	16
9.10	62	30	28	26	24	24	23	22	22	21	20	20	19	19	18	17	16
10.0	64	31	29	27	25	24	24	23	22	21	21	20	20	19	19	18	17
10.3	65	32	29	27	26	25	24	23	23	22	21	21	20	19	19	18	17
10.7	67	33	30	28	26	26	25	24	23	23	22	21	20	20	19	18	17
10.10	68	33	31	29	27	26	25	25	24	23	22	22	21	20	20	19	18
11.0	70	34	32	30	28	27	26	25	24	24	23	22	22	21	30	19	18
11.3	71	35	32	30	28	27	26	26	25	24	23	23	22	21	21	20	19
11.7	73	36	33	31	29	28	27	26	26	25	24	23	23	22	21	20	19
11.10	74	36	34	32	30	29	28	27	26	25	24	24	23	22	22	21	20
12.0	76	37	35	32	30	29	28	28	27	26	25	24	24	23	22	21	20
12.3	78	38	35	33	31	30	29	28	27	26	26	25	24	23	23	22	20
12.7	79	39	36	34	32	31	30	29	28	27	26	25	25	24	23	22	21
12.10	81	39	37	34	32	31	30	29	28	27	27	26	25	24	24	22	21
13.0	83	40	38	35	33	32	31	30	29	28	27	26	26	25	24	23	22
13.3	84	41	38	36	33	32	31	30	29	29	28	27	26	25	25	23	22
13.7	86	42	39	36	34	33	32	31	30	29	28	27	27	26	25	24	23
13.10	87	43	40	37	35	34	33	31	31	30	29	28	27	26	26	24	23
14.0	89	43	41	38	35	34	33	32	31	30	29	28	28	27	26	25	23
14.3	90	44	41	38	36	35	34	33	32	31	30	29	28	27	27	25	24
14.7	92	45	42	39	37	36	34	33	32	31	30	30	29	28	27	26	24
14.10	93	46	43	40	37	36	35	34	33	32	31	30	29	28	27	26	25
15.0	95	47	43	41	38	37	36	34	33	32	31	31	30	29	28	27	25
15.3	97	47	44	41	39	37	36	35	34	33	32	31	30	29	28	27	25
15.7	98	48	45	42	39	38	37	36	35	34	33	32	31	30	29	27	26
15.10	100	49	46	43	40	39	37	36	35	34	33	32	31	30	29	28	26
16.0	102	50	46	43	41	39	38	37	36	35	34	33	32	31	30	28	27
16.3	103	50	47	44	41	40	39	37	36	35	34	33	32	31	30	29	27

UNDERSTANDING YOUR BASAL METABOLIC RATE

So now you know all about your BMI, your Body Mass Index and through this you now know what is the correct weight for you and more importantly you know exactly what weight you are going to attain. Yes, another goal planned.

Now we come to your BMR, your basal metabolic rate. Your BMR is the rate at which your body burns calories when at rest, over a 24 hour period.

An approxiamate but surprisingly accurate calculation of your BMR is simply:

Multiply your weight in Kg by 92.4 or in lbs by 10.0

Eg 80 Kg by 92.4 = 7392 Kj or 1760 Cal

Or lbs 176 by 10.0 = 1760 Cal or 7392 Kj

Of course your average daily burn of calories is going to be more than 1760, after all you can't lay flat on your back every day for 24 hours.

Now we establish your activity level and multiply by the factor below. We will work in Kg's and calories for simplicity.

Low   by 1.3

Mediam by 1.4

High   by 1.5

Very High by 1.7

Eg : An office worker at a low level of activity weighing 70 Kg's

70 by 92.4 = 6468 Kj's (divide by 4.2 for Cal's) = 1540 Cal's

Multiplied by 1.3 = 2002 Calories (your average daily energy burn)

You can see how your daily calorie intake must be under this to lose weight.

I will explain more later on in the exercise prescription section how exercise and increases in lean muscle mass can increase your BMR.

HOW AM I GOING TO LOSE IT ?

Firstly please remember the Golden Rule of weight loss.

For weight loss to occur the daily calorie intake must be less than the daily energy expenditure.

You are going to reduce your daily calorie intake, increase your daily calorie output, without going hungry, without having to use huge amounts of willpower and without the tedious job of counting calories, all whilst maintaining your required balance of vitamins and minerals.

You are going to lose at least ½ Kilo per week until your desired weight is reached.

1 Kg Fat = approx 8000 Calories.

To lose ½ Kilo per week you are going to reduce your calorie intake by at least 4000 per week = approx 570 per day.

Example : If you are 70 Kg & your optimal weight is 60 Kg you will reach your target weight in 20 weeks at most, many will attain the 60 Kg goal a lot sooner depending on factors such as diligence, age, gender, joint soundness and general levels of activity, oh, and don't forget good old Genetics.

You are not going to have to worry about such things as the number of calories or kilojoules, grams of carbohydrate, protein or fat per Kg of body weight or vague terms such as 'more of this group' or 'a percentage of these types of foods'. How boring and complicated. No, all this has been meticulously sorted for you so relax and enjoy.

EXERCISE

Yes, I know you can't wait to start working on that muscle tone, getting stuck into your fat-burning cardio programs and blissfully stretching those tight muscles back to their full flexible length.

Ok, now let's have a look at the overall situation here and what ground we have covered to date. Remembering that it is all about the big four, Balance, Clarity, Direction and Discipline, we will look at where you are now.

- You appreciate the numerous benefits of exercise
- You understand the basic facts of sustainable dieting
- You now clearly understand the **Glycaemic Index**
- You know the importance of keeping records
- You have your full shopping list in alphabetical order
- You have the confidence that all your foods have been fully researched and have been selected on their GI values, Fibre, Sugar, Carbohydrate, Protein, Fat and Calories (amounts & type)
- You fully understand your BMI (Body Mass Index) and have estimated what weight is right for you
- You know all about your BMR (Basal Metabolic Rate) and what your average daily calorie burn equates to according to your energy levels
- You are aware of how much weight (minimum) you are going to lose each week
- You are fully aware of **how** this weight loss occurs
- You have sufficient recipes to begin your new eating program.

If I was you I would be feeling quietly confident at this point and quite proud of myself.

Next I would like you to look at your physical condition prior to engaging in exercise by following my advice on the next page.

The exercises range from the very basic through to the intermediate stages. Even though the exercise and dietary aspects apply to anyone it is assumed that the majority of participants are overweight and are neither regular nor experienced with exercise routines.

Normally in a face to face situation with a new client (personal training client) I have a general health & lifestyle questionnaire of which the client answers numerous questions relating to their health, exercise history, their goals, and medical history (both past and present) So I have included the questions below that are of major concern. If you answer yes to any of them I strongly recommend that you see your doctor or relevant health professional prior to beginning any of the exercise programs.

- Have you any heart condition (past or present) that you are aware of ?
- Do you suffer from asthma ?
- Is your blood pressure more than 140/90 ?
- Do you suffer from diabetes ?
- Are you taking any prescribed medication ?
- Do you ever suffer from dizziness or fainting ?
- Are you over 45 years of age ?
- Are you pregnant ?
- Do you suffer any back pain ?
- Are you currently carrying any injury ?
- Do you suffer from epilepsy ?

Now I assume that either you have answered no to all these questions or you have answered yes to one or more of them and have seen your doctor or appropriate medical professional and have been cleared to begin your exercise.

I would like to emphasize here that no matter how mobile or overweight you may be, the gradual build-up of your cardio, muscular strength and flexibility are extremely important. As well as burning up calories they have the added benefits of preparing you for higher intensities later on through strengthening your bones, ligaments and increasing your aerobic capacity.

BASIC FITNESS ASSESSMENT

YOUR HEART RATE

Your pulse or heart rate is what will form the basis of your level of exercise intensity for your aerobic conditioning.

Maximal heart rate (MHR) is the highest heart rate a person can attain during heavy exercise. To work at this maximum heart rate is both dangerous and unnecessary, so we work to a specific formulae (known as the Karvonen Formulae) which is 220 – your age.

As we age our maximum heart rate becomes lower, so it is of even greater importance to monitor the heart rate of an older person, as it is for an un-conditioned or un-fit person. All work performed will be at a percentage of your maximum heart rate as shown below. Your resting heart rate (RHR) is the rate at which your heart beats per minute when at rest.

Example for a 40 year old

220 – 40 (age) = 180 (MHR)

For an un-fit or overweight person I am recommending that we begin working at 70% of your maximum heart rate, i.e : 126 bpm.

I find an easy way of working out your percentage (without a calculator) is to simply divide the 180 (MHR) and the percentage by 10 and multiply e.g :

70% of 180 = 7 times 18 = 126

50% of 180 = 5 times 18 = 90

A wonderful tool to utilize, particularly when you are starting out is a Heart Rate Monitor. These are available at all good sports stores and a decent one will set you back about $200. Otherwise calculate your heart rate by counting your pulse rate over 15 seconds and multiply by 4 for one minute. At the wrist with index and middle fingers (not your thumb)

Setting and continually attaining your goals is what keeps you on track. Now we are going to do some basic fitness assessment tests of which are great to give you an idea of your ability and limitations at this early stage. Make sure you keep a record of each test so you can compare notes at regular intervals.

RESTING HEART RATE

Have a clock with a second hand next to your bed. On waking take your heart rate at the wrist either for 15 seconds multiplied by 4 or for the full minute. This is your resting heart rate. This is a good habit to get into as it helps you to become more confident in taking your heart rate at other times and it can be very motivating to see your heart rate dropping as you become fitter. It is nice to know the old heart doesn't have to work so hard as it used to.

THE STEP TEST

Find a step approx 45cm high and fairly solid to comfortably take your weight when standing freely on it. With your watch or clock in view, begin stepping up and down from the step, left foot up, left foot down, right foot up, right foot down for 5 minutes at a reasonable pace. On completion immediately take your heart rate at 1 minute, 2 minutes and 3 minutes (recording times) Doing this test at a later date will show a much lower heart rate proving your increasing fitness and aerobic capacity.

ABDOMINAL STRENGTH AND ENDURANCE

Laying on the floor with knees up and arms straight out in the horizontal position, lift your shoulders off the ground in a crunch position until your wrists cover your knees. Do as many as you can in one minute, or 30 seconds if this is not possible. Through your pilates and yoga moves later on you will notice huge improvements in your core-strength.

EXERCISE FACTS

- Exercise will increase your cardio-vascular fitness
- Help prevent heart disease and stroke
- Assist with rectifying blood pressure problems
- Reduce the risk of diabetes & osteoporosis
- Improve your bone density
- Help maintain sustainable weight loss
- Build and maintain lean muscle mass
- Increase strength
- Help attain your desired body shape
- Increase the strength of your tendons & ligaments
- Assist in maintaining good posture
- Enable you to live a long, healthy & rewarding life
- Increase overall energy levels
- Improve mental well-being
- Boost your self esteem
- Reduce anxiety & depression
- Help develop a deep inner confidence
- Help prevent alzheimers through neural genesis
- Increase your daily productivity capabilities
- Assist the body's nutritional and hormonal balances
- Keep you looking young and vibrant
- Reduce your resting heart rate
- Help you sleep more soundly

EXERCISE

Your exercise programs are a balanced combination of Cardio, Resistance training and Stretching.

As your personal trainer (me) is not physically with you I have laid out balanced, full body programs that will attain the desired benefits of increased strength, flexibility and aerobic fitness. There are many reasons why it is absolutely impossible to prescribe exactly the same exercise routines for everyone. Some of these reasons include a client's level of fitness, their age, available time, joint problems, medical reasons, past injuries and even likes and dislikes. It doesn't worry me at all if a particular client would prefer not to run, as I will obtain a similar training effect through swimming or bike work. The exercise chart at the beginning of the exercise prescription section is for you to photocopy and keep regular records of your work. Following shortly are detailed descriptions together with pictures of all the exercises you will be performing.

CARDIO AND AEROBIC CONDITIONING

You know all about your maximum heart rate and how to take your pulse, so do this often in the early stages. Later on you know from experience what rate you are working at. The cardio work I have prescribed revolves around walking, swimming, running, bike riding and classes. The level of intensity rises gradually and again please keep in mind that flexibility is paramount in that you may have to adjust either up or down to suit your individual capabilities. This type of training increases heart and lung capacities as the body draws steadily on it's reserves of fuel, e.g fat. In a fairly short space of time you will notice thrilling improvements in the way you feel, particularly increased energy levels. Some of you may prefer group exercise classes, play team games or go mountain climbing on weekends, these all count as part of your cardio exercise routine. An interesting comparison is with running and swimming, and when performed at equal intensities (equal heart rates) a 5 Km run is equivalent to a 1 Km swim.

STRENGTH AND RESISTANCE TRAINING

The benefits of resistance training are well documented. Some of the better known benefits include maintaining bone density (preventing osteoporosis) increasing your strength and helping to keep good posture for life. Some benefits you may not know include, increases in your metabolic rate (assisting the fat-burning effect) it maintains muscle mass of which diminishes with age, and is responsible for changes in body composition and muscle tone.

A number of my female clients often ask, will weights make me bulky ? Creating body mass or bulking up is quite an intentional thing to do and you must train specifically for it, plus it is pretty much restricted to the guys with all that testosterone, so don't worry girls, your light weights, plenty of repetitions and lack of testosterone won't allow you to do it.

In performing the prescribed exercises, all you require are three items, a fitball, a pair of dumbbells and a resistance tube. The resistance tube is a rubber tube with a handle on each end and they come in a mediam or strong resistance. Before you purchase it ask if you can try it out to decide which resistance suits you. Standing tall, slip the tube under your feet with handles facing palm forward. Now flex your forearms up toward your shoulder performing a bicep curl. If you can do 15 repetitions easily and feel as though you can do more it's too light, go for the stronger one. I will go through all exercises using the resistance tube later on. Again, with the dumbbells ask for assistance and if you can perform 15 repetitions of the bicep curl easily, go for the next size up. Remember that your strength will improve very quickly and you will probably require a heavier set later on. With regard to the fitball, go for a good quality one, usually the more pronounced the ribs are the stronger and better quality the ball is.

STRETCHING

Stretching is a vital part of your program often neglected by many. Exercise actually has the effect of tightening your muscles, so it is of great importance while your muscles are warm to stretch them after exercise returning them to their original lengths. This will prevent the risk of injury and stiffness and maintain good flexibility. See pics of all your required stretches and remember to hold each stretch for at least 30 seconds.

EXERCISE PROGRAMS

All your exercises are programmed on a daily basis covering a three month period. Each of you will find your own level and stay flexible with regard to your resistance, number of repetitions and cardio intensity.

The reasons for this flexible approach include :

- Your exercise history / capability / experience
- Your general physical fitness
- Male or female
- Past or present injuries
- Medical considerations
- Your preferences
- Training specifically for particular sports or goals
- Progressive overload, where you are naturally going to be improving all the time, it is necessary that all facets of your programs increase in intensity as you attain your goals.

Many of you will not have any exercise experience at all. Some of you will be classified as obese where any movement at all is difficult for you. A number of you will have group exercise experience, but are overweight and some of you may be recovering from a lengthy illness. There will also be some of you of whom are reasonably fit with an acceptable body shape but wish to improve, (these people usually don't have a problem with goal setting) So you can see the benefits of this flexible approach.

Exercise programs are designed for 3 levels of intensity, Low, Mediam and High. They are also clearly separated into Resistance and Cardio components. I strongly advise you to begin under what you think you may be able to handle and work your way up, a solid preparation is very important as you strengthen your muscles, ligaments and joints in preparation for higher intensities later on.

Please don't forget to complete the full stretching routine after every session.

Your prescribed resistance exercises will be performed at a nominated number of repetitions and sets.

A repetition is the completion of an exercise from start to finish.

The number of repetitions is the number times you perform that exercise.

The number of sets is the number of times that the total number of those repetitions are performed.

And finally, remember to breathe out as you perform your exercises and breathe in as you return to the start.

CHEST PRESS

The chest press is a great compound exercise working the pectoral muscles, triceps and shoulders. It is often performed in the gym and commonly known as the bench press. Below are two ways of performing this exercise, with the resistance tube and dumbells on the fitball.

CHEST PRESS (RESISTANCE TUBE)

- Stand with your feet hip width apart, knees slightly bent and your back nice and straight.
- Pass the resistance tube over your head and across your upper back while holding the handles in an overhand grip as pictured.
- With your hands in line with your chest, breathe in and push away from your chest, extending your arms while breathing out.
- Breathing in, return to the starting position and repeat.

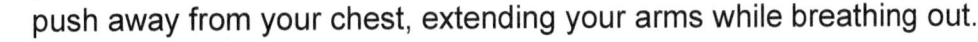

CHEST PRESS (FITBALL)

- Grasp the dumbbells in both hands and siton the fitball.
- Now lean back onto the fitball and walk
- yourself forward until your shoulders and neck are comfortably supported on the ball. As pictured, make sure your body is nice and straight with your lower legs perpendicular.

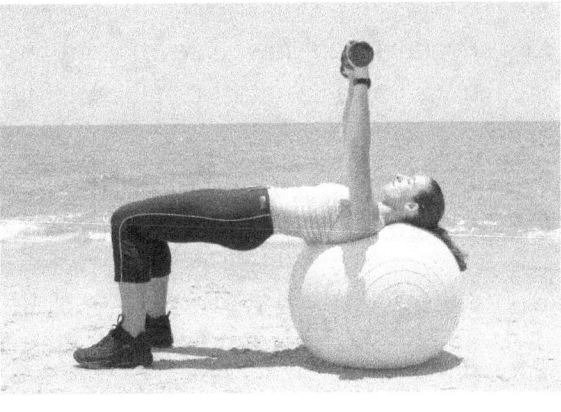

- With your upper arms horizontal, take a breath and extend your arms up with a full range of movement, bringing the dumbbells fairly close together at the top of the movement.
- Taking a breath return to the starting position and repeat.

THE PUSH-UP

The old faithful push-up, don't you love it? Great for your chest, shoulders and upper arms. This is one exercise that you can do anywhere, drop and give me 20! Following are 3 levels of push-up which allows the client (you) to progress gradually with an increase in intensity.

PUSH-UP (KNEES) Also known as the 'Box' push-up.

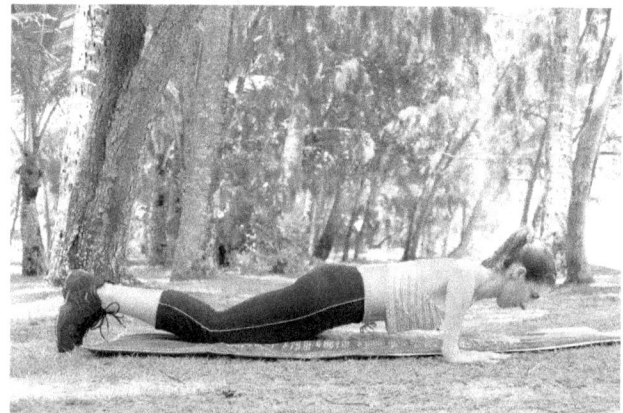

- Kneel on the floor with your feet together or slightly spread with your knees under your hips.
- Place your hands under your shoulders, a bit wider than shoulder width apart with your fingers pointing forwards.
- Keep your body weight distributed over your hands, and your abs contracted with a nice flat back.
- Breathing in, lower down until the elbows reach 90 degrees, now push back up to the start position while breathing out.

EXTENDED 'BOX' PUSH-UP (KNEES)

- As for above except now you lift your lower legs to 90 degrees. This increases the weight on your shoulders and arms.

THE PUSH-UP

- Place your hands under your shoulders, a bit wider than shoulder width apart with your fingers pointing forwards.
- Keep your body and legs straight, with your feet about hip-width apart and up on your toes.
- Keeping your head in line with your spine, breathe in and lower yourself down so that your arms are at 90 degrees.
- Now, keeping those abs tight, push back up to the start breathing out as you finish.

BENT – OVER RAISE (RESISTANCE TUBE)

An exercise that will give definition (tone) in your upper back and shoulders (posterior deltoids)

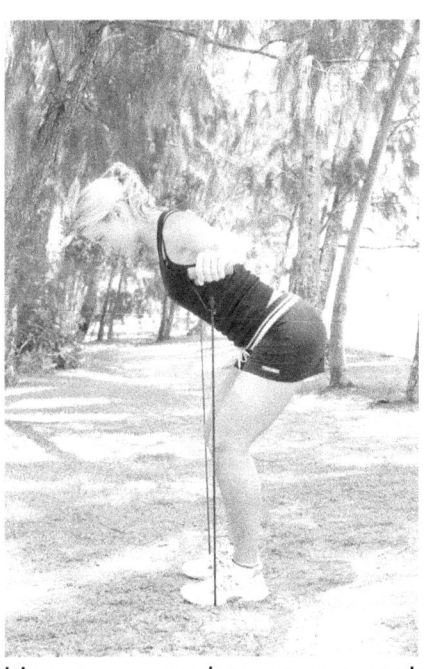

- Stand in the centre of the resistance tube with your feet about hip-width apart, knees slightly bent and your back nice and straight.
- Wrap the resistance tube once around each foot (this shortens it for you and increases the resistance) Taking a handle in each hand, bend forward from the waist holding the handles below the hips.
- With your arms slightly bent, open them out and lift up to shoulder height slowly returning to the start, making sure you keep your neck muscles relaxed.

PEC-FLY (RESISTANCE TUBE)

An effective exercise for the chest and is complimentary to the chest press and the push up.

- At roughly waist height, find a pole or railing and wrap your resistance tube around it a couple of times.
- About arms length from the pole, stand with your legs hip-width apart knees slightly bent and your back nice and straight.
- Now grasp both the resistance tube's handles in one hand, keeping the arm slightly bent.
- Without moving your body at all bring the hand around towards you to the centre of your chest. Repeat your required reps and switch to the other arm.

TRICEPS

Now girls, I know you want to tighten up those loose bits that tend to hang down at the back of the arms. The triceps are a group of muscles at the back of the arm and are used to straighten the arm. Below are 2 methods available to you in exercising your triceps.

OVERHEAD TRICEP EXTENSION (RESISTANCE TUBE)

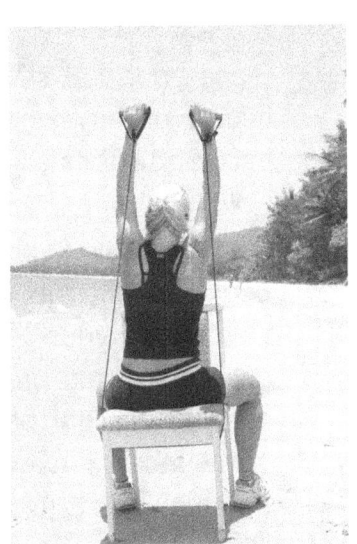

- Lay the exercise tube either on the floor or across a chair and sit on it grasping both handles behind the neck.
- With your elbows pointed towards the ceiling extend your arms close to the side of your head and just forward of your shoulders.
- Return to starting position and repeat, remembering to breathe out as you complete each repetition.

TRICEP KICKBACK (DUMBELL)

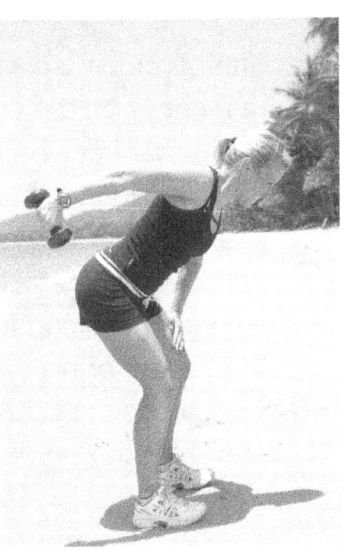

- Grasp a dumbbell in your right hand and take a step forward, slightly bending at both knees.
- Keeping your back straight, bend forward from the waist while placing your left hand on your left knee as a support.
- With your right arm bent at 90 degrees press the upper part of your arm against your side and straighten your arm breathing out as you complete the movement.
- Inhaling, return the arm to the start position and complete the required amount of reps before changing arms.

SHOULDER PRESS

The shoulder press is fantastic for upper arm and shoulder definition, working the deltoids and the triceps. Three ways you can perform this exercise are laid out below.

RESISTANCE TUBE

- Place your feet shoulder width apart in the middle of the exercise tube with a straight back and knees slightly bent.
- Hold the handles at shoulder height with the tube behind your arms.
- Begin with the elbows level with your chest, then press your arms up over your head until your arms are almost fully extended, keeping a slight bend in your elbows and palms facing forward.
- Breathe in on returning to start and repeat.

SEATED DUMBELL PRESS

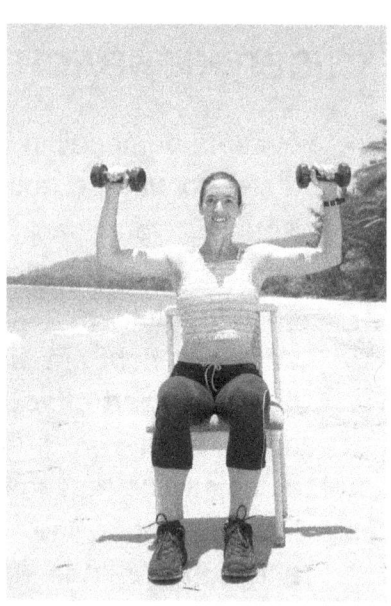

- Find a good solid chair and place your dumbbells on the floor in front of it.
- Sit at the front part of the chair with your back facing the chairs back.
- Pick up your dumbbells with an overhand grip and lift them to shoulder height, with your palms facing forward.
- Inhale and press your arms to an extended vertical position breathing out as you go and keeping your elbows soft (slightly bent)

SEATED DUMBELL PRESS (FITBALL)

- Sit on fitball with back straight and feet flat on the deck with dumbells in front of you.
- Complete the exercise as with seated dumbbell press.

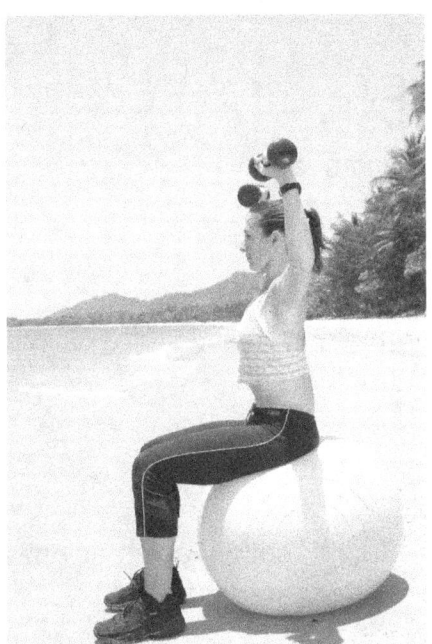

LATERAL RAISE

The lateral raise is a really worthwhile exercise as it primarily targets the medial deltoids, (middle / top section of the shoulder) promoting shape and strength throughout the upper arm and shoulder region. Following are 3 methods of performing the same exercise.

RESISTANCE TUBE

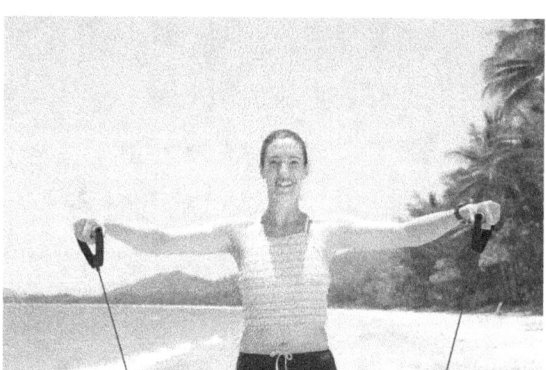

- With your feet hip-width apart stand in the centre of the resistance tube, keeping your knees slightly bent.
- Begin with your arms by your sides, your abs contracted and your back straight.
- Slowly raise your arms to horizontal (shoulder) level, keeping your back straight, palms facing downwards and your torso nice and still, then lower back to start position.

STANDING (DUMBELLS)

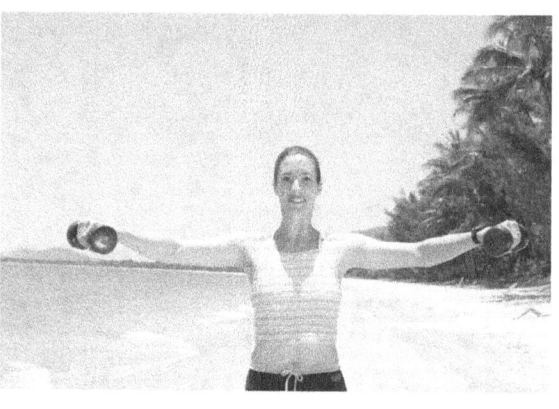

- With a straight back stand with your feet hip-width apart and knees slightly bent.
- With your arms hanging by your sides, holding a dumbbell in each hand, raise the dumbbells to shoulder level remembering to keep your elbows slightly bent.
- Return to starting position and repeat.

FITBALL (DUMBELLS)

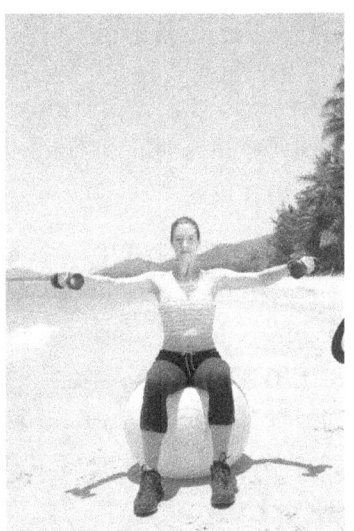

- Taking a dumbbell in each hand sit on the ball with your back straight and your feet flat on the floor.
- With your arms hanging by your sides, raise the dumbbells to shoulder level and return to start, remembering to keep those abs nice and tight.

UPRIGHT ROW

The upright row promotes shoulder shape and strength with intense work on the trapezius (upper back / shoulder area) and secondary work on the biceps.

RESISTANCE TUBE

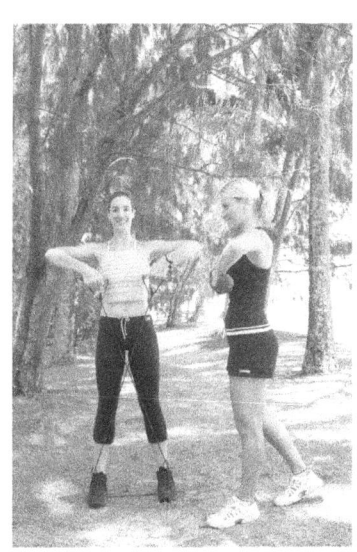

- Keeping your back straight and knees slightly bent, place your feet in the centre of the resistance tube.
- Cross the handles over in front of you keeping your palms facing inwards.
- Pull the handles up to chin height lifting your elbows as high as possible, breathing out as you complete the movement.
- Breathing in slowly lower back to the starting position.

SEATED ROW

The seated row is without doubt one exercise no one should leave out of their routine. It is a real back builder, working the lats, rear delts and biceps just to name a few.

As you bring your shoulder blades (scapulae) together you work your traps and rhomboids. And if that's not enough to convince you, as you return to the starting position under load, you are actually stretching your lats (latissimus dorsi)

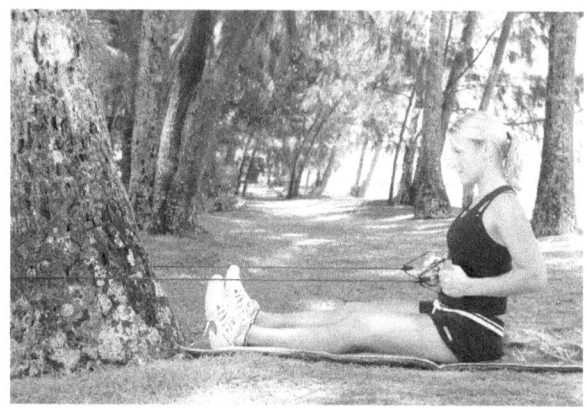

- Sit on the floor and place the exercise tube at the soles of both feet. Now wrap the tube once around each foot and adjust until even length.
- Keeping your legs together, your knees slightly bent and your back straight, take the grips of the exercise tube with palms facing inwards.
- Keeping your hands low and your arms close to your body, pull the handles toward you until our shoulder blades come together.
- Slowly return to the start breathing in as you go.

THE ONE ARM ROW

The one arm row is a great exercise for the back, upper arm and shoulder region. Below are two examples of performing this exercise, with the resistance tube and a flat bench.

RESISTANCE TUBE

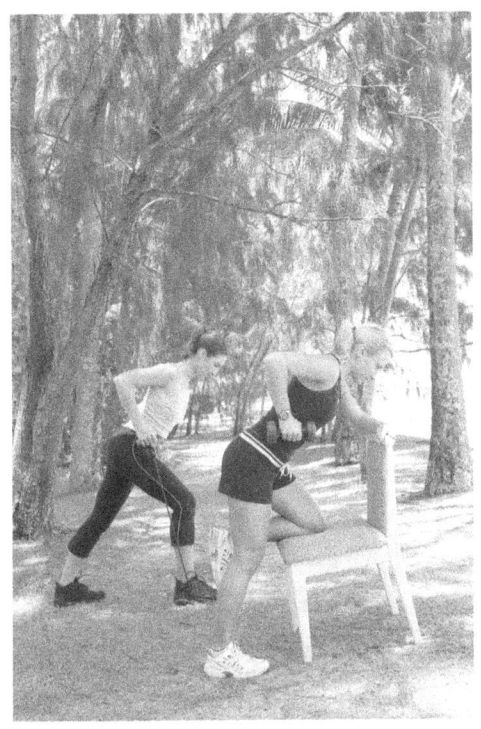

- Secure the resistance tube to the floor with with one foot about one third the way along the tube.
- With the other foot take a good step back behind you, keeping the leg straight and the heel flat to the floor.
- Allow the long end of the tube to lay on the floor as you grasp the short end, keeping your arm relaxed, with the other arm resting on your hip or thigh.
- Aim to keep your body at 45 degrees with a nice straight line running from head to heel, making sure that your front knee stays above and behind your toes and your hips are facing straight ahead.
- Exhaling, pull the handle of the resistance tube up toward your chest until your elbow is at right angles and close to your body.
- Focus on keeping the body stable, with a straight back and relaxed shoulders. Return slowly to starting position and repeat on the other arm.

ONE ARM ROW (DUMBELL)

- On a flat bench (approx 18 in / 45 cm high) grasp the dumbbell with palm facing inwards, while resting the opposite hand and knee on the bench.
- Keeping your elbow back, bring the dumbbell up as high as possible exhaling as you complete the movement.

BICEP CURL

As with most resistance exercises there are many variations of which re-distribute the work to different muscles. The bicep curl is no exception, however at this stage we are only concentrating on the basic movements. Following are three methods of performing this exercise.

RESISTANCE TUBE

- Take a handle in each hand and stand in the middle of the resistance tube with your feet hip-width apart and knees slightly bent.
- With your elbows slightly bent and your arms by your sides, making sure your palms face upwards.
- Lift (curl) both arms toward your chest until your hands are level with your shoulders, making sure that your back is straight and your elbows are tucked in to your sides.
- At the top of the movement contract the bicep to increase the effectiveness, then slowly return to the start remembering your breathing.

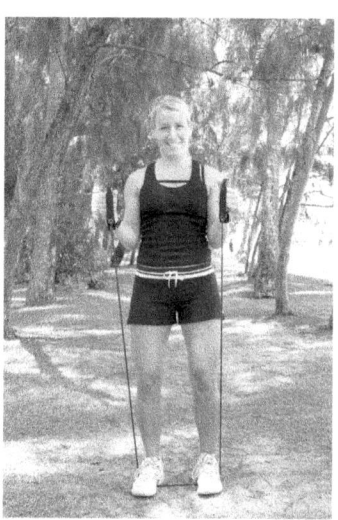

FITBALL (DUMBBELL CURLS)

- Sit on the ball with your feet flat on the floor and the dumbbells in front of you.
- With a dumbbell in each hand hanging at your sides, and your palms facing inward, raise one dumbbell turning the palm up as you bring it to shoulder level, lower as you repeat with the other arm.

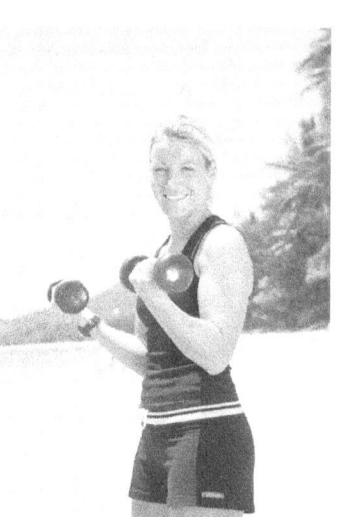

ALTERNATE DUMBBELL CURLS (STANDING)

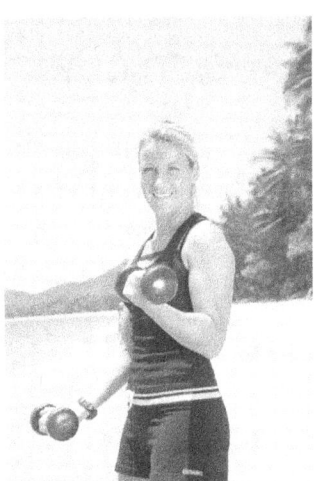

- Stand with feet hip-width apart and knees slightly bent with a dumbbell in each hand.
- With palms facing inward, raise one dumbbell turning the palm up as you bring it to shoulder level, lower as you repeat with the other arm.
- Flex the bicep at the top of the movement to increase intensity.

HAMMER CURL (RESISTANCE TUBE)

The hammer curl is a variation of the bicep curl and includes the outer part of your bicep promoting shape and tone.

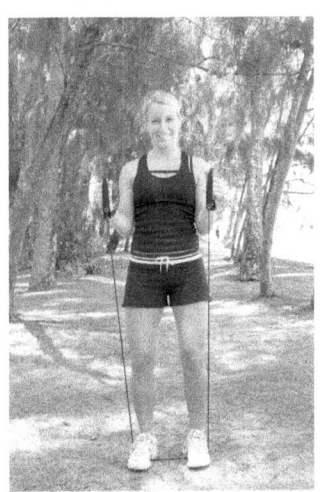

- Stand in the middle of the resistance tube with feet about hip-width apart, knees slightly bent and back straight.
- Contract your abs as you grasp a handle in each hand with your palms facing inwards (thumbs to the top)
- Keeping your elbows tucked in to your sides, lift the handles towards your shoulders,contracting the bicep at the end of the movement.

HAMMER CURL (STANDING / DUMBBELLS)

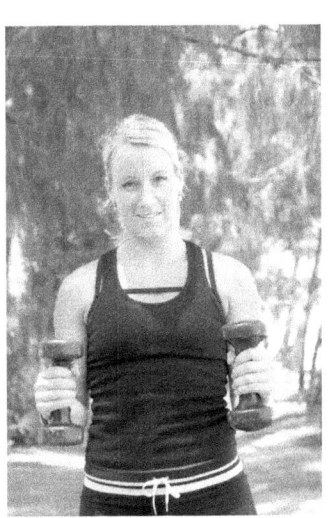

- Stand tall with feet about hip-width apart, knees slightly bent and back nice and straight.
- Grasp a dumbbell in each hand with your palms facing inwards. Now curl the dumbbells toward your shoulders.
- Return to the starting position and repeat for the required amount of repetitions.

HAMMER CURL VARIATIONS

- The hammer curl, using dumbbells can also be performed sitting on a fitball. An excellent variation is lifting each dumbbell alternately instead of together (the alternate dumbbell curl)

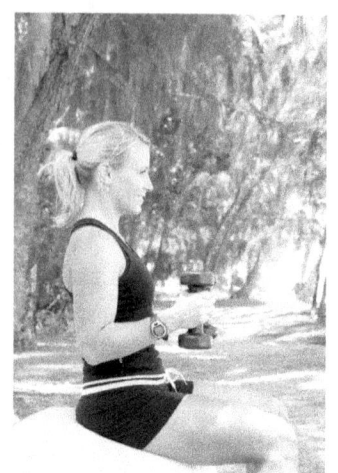

SINGLE LEG SQUAT

Great for the bum and thighs. May require some practice to perfect, as good balance is required.

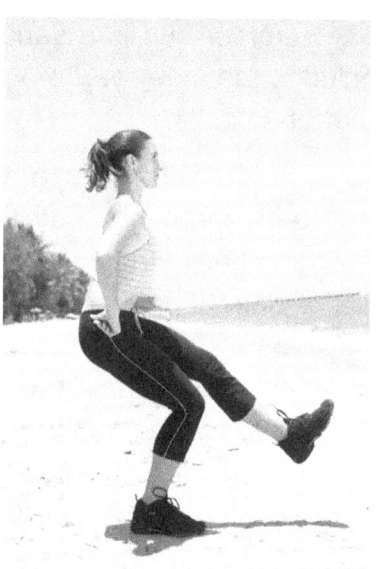

- Take up your standard starting posture, with feet hip-width apart and your knees slightly bent, make sure you keep your abs contracted whilst keeping your back straight.
- Place your hands on your hips and raise one leg straight out in front of you, while keeping the heel approx (6in / 150 mm) off the floor.
- As with the normal squat, imagine that you are going to sit on a chair, controlling the movement while maintaining a good straight back.
- Come down under full control to about 90 degrees (no less) then raise yourself back to the starting position. Perform the required number of reps before swapping over to the other leg.

SQUAT (RESISTANCE TUBE)

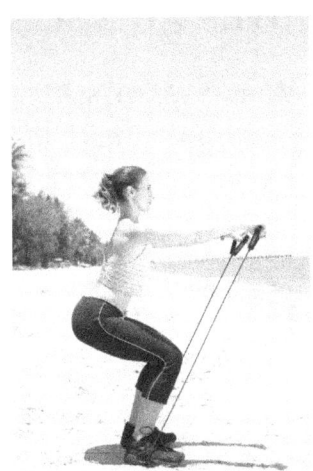

- Stand in the centre of the tube with your feet hip-width apart, knees slightly bent and back straight.
- Holding the handles at shoulder level, lower your torso as though you are about to sit in a chair.
- Keeping abs contracted and heels down, come down to about 90 degrees, approx parallel to the floor, breathing in as you go.
- Breathing out return to starting position and repeat.

POWER LUNGE

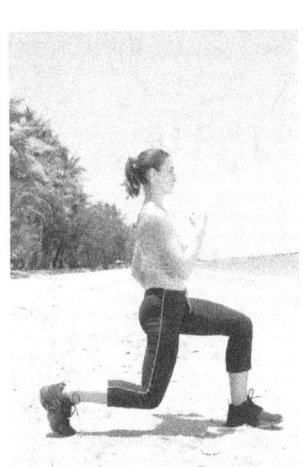

- Stand upright, feet hip-width apart, facing forward with your hands on your hips.
- As you take a good step forwards, lower your body making sure that your front knee doesn't move past your ankle.
- Now, spring back to the starting position keeping your body steady and push back through the heel of the front foot.
- Complete the required number of reps and switch to the other leg.

LUNGE (RESISTANCE TUBE)

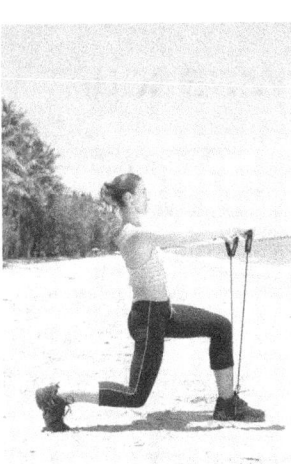

- Take a good step forward placing the middle of the tube under the arch of your front foot.
- Hold the handles at your hip or shoulder level (depending on what resistance you require)
- Lower your body, lifting the heel of your rear foot as you go, making sure that your front knee doesn't move past your ankle.
- Complete the required amount of repetitions and switch over to the other leg and repeat.

STEP AND SQUAT

Wow ! we're starting to work now. The step squat increases the intensity on the working leg and creates more work on the inner thigh and bum.

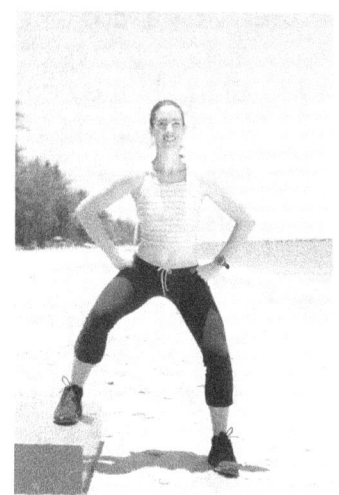

- Find a stair or step about 12 inches (30 cm) high.
- As you step down off the step bend your knees as you assume the squat position, leaning forwards slightly as you come down, making sure you keep your heels on the deck.
- Return to the starting position noting how you now use the strength of the other leg.
- Face the other way and repeat.

STEP UP

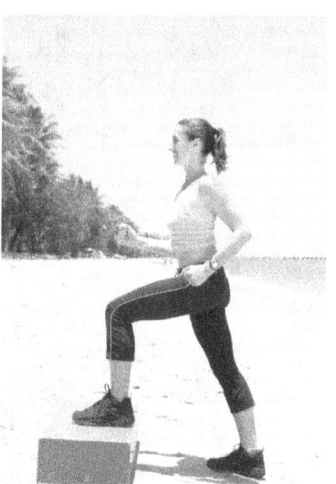

- Find a step at least 18in (45cm) high.
- Facing the step place the leading foot flat on the step.
- Step up with the other foot making sure that you keep your head and neck relaxed and your back straight.
- Step back down with your leading foot first.
- Repeat with your other leg going up first.

WIDE SQUAT

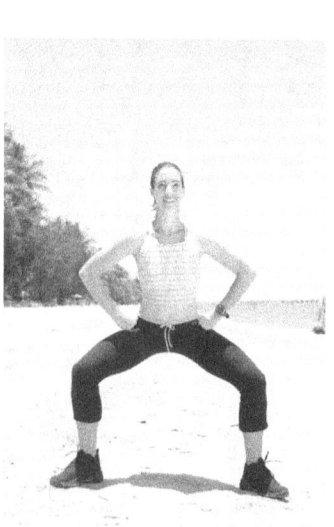

- With your hands on your hips stand with your feet just a bit wider than shoulder width apart and your toes pointing out.
- Bending your knees as though you are about to sit in a chair, come down to almost 90 degrees making sure to breathe in as you come down.
- Breathing out, raise your body back to the start.

OUTER THIGH / HIP (ABDUCTION)

SIDE LEG LIFTS (RESISTANCE TUBE)

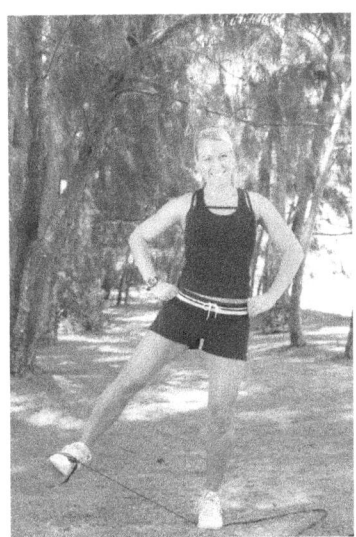

- Standing with knees slightly bent and back straight, place one foot in one handle of the resistance tube.
- Now place the opposite foot on the tube about (6in / 150cm) away from the looped foot.
- Lift the looped foot out to the side as far as you can, pause and return to starting position.
- Complete required repetitions and change to other leg.
- Do not lean over at the hip and work within your comfort range.

FLOOR HIP ABDUCTIONS

- Lie on your side keeping your head and shoulders in line, using your forearm for support.
- Keeping your leg straight, lift the leg to an angle of about 60 degrees off the floor.
- Return to starting position and repeat.

INNER THIGH PRESS / ADDUCTION (RESISTANCE TUBE)

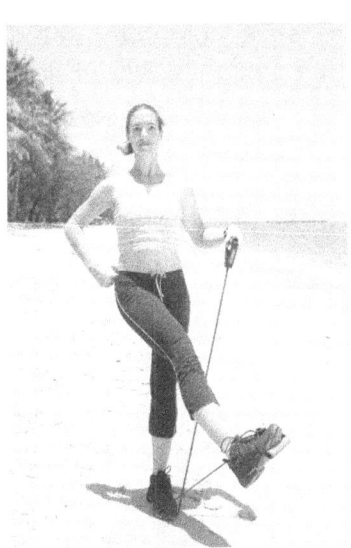

- Insert one foot in a tube handle, then stand on the tube with the other foot, about (6in / 150mm) from the looped foot while holding the free handle in the other hand.
- Standing tall, find your balance before pushing the right foot forward and across your body keeping the toes close to the floor.
- Reach the extent of your movement without allowing your hips to shift out of alignment, then return to start.
- Complete required amount of reps and switch legs.

SIDE LUNGE

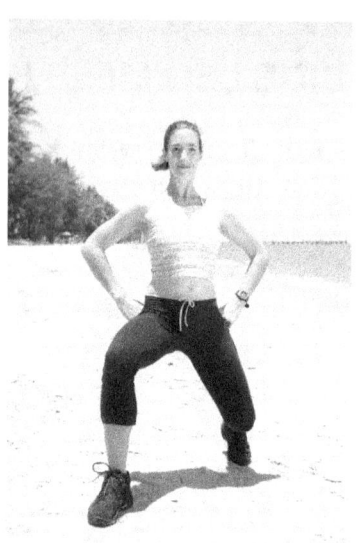

- Standing with your feet hip-width apart, knees slightly bent and your hands on your hips.
- Facing with your hips to the front take a good sized step forward at 45 degrees, planting your foot a good step ahead of your back foot.
- Keeping your body upright and your abs contracted, bend both knees, bringing the front knee directly over your front foot, without going past the tongue of your shoe.
- Come down so that your front knee is at about 90 degrees and your back knee is approx (6in / 150mm) from the deck. Placing the weight on to the heel of your front foot will intensify the work on the gluts (bum)

KNEE RAISE

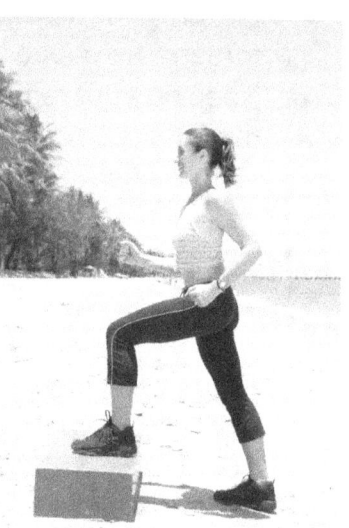

This exercise is tougher than it looks and fantastic for good looking legs.

- Find a step about (45cm / 18in) high or slightly less. Facing the step, keep your back nice and straight with your hands on your hips.
- Keeping one foot on the floor, place the other foot on the step.
- Now, step up with the other foot, but instead of placing it on the step, lift it up, raising your knee to hip height.
- Lower your leg so that both feet are on the step, then step back to the floor with your leading leg first.

SQUAT (RESISTANCE TUBE)

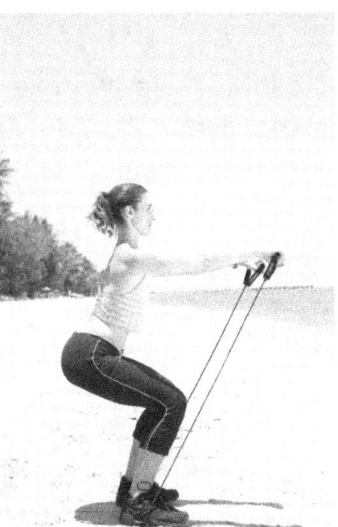

- Stand in the centre of the tube, with a straight back, knees slightly bent, and feet about hip-width apart.
- Grasp the handles and hold at either hip or shoulder level (depending on what resistance you require) and sit back into your hips.
- Lower yourself into a squat position (as though you are about to sit in a chair) until your thighs are almost parallel to the floor.
- Breathing out, return to the standing position, keeping your heels down and your abdominals contracted.

OBLIQUES

Following are two exercises for the obliques. The obliques (muscles at the side of your abs) are often neglected in exercise programs, but work here will really compliment that waistline.

SIDE BENDS (RESISTANCE TUBE)

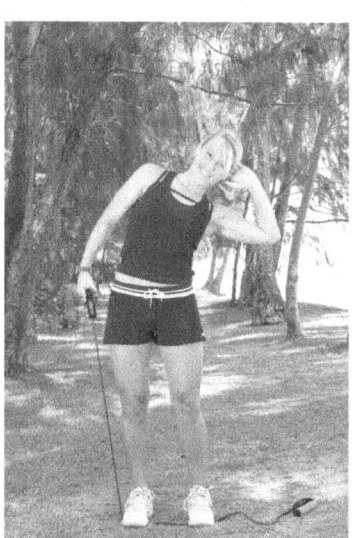

- Stand in the middle of the resistance tube making sure that your feet are about hip-width apart, with your knees slightly bent and your back nice and straight.
- Grasp the handle (leave the other one on the floor) keeping the arm straight down beside your body and contract your abs.
- Now bend away from the handle you are holding and return to starting position.
- Lean over to a comfortable range, without aggravation to the lower back. You can adjust the position of your foot on the tube to alter the resistance.

OBLIQUE CRUNCH

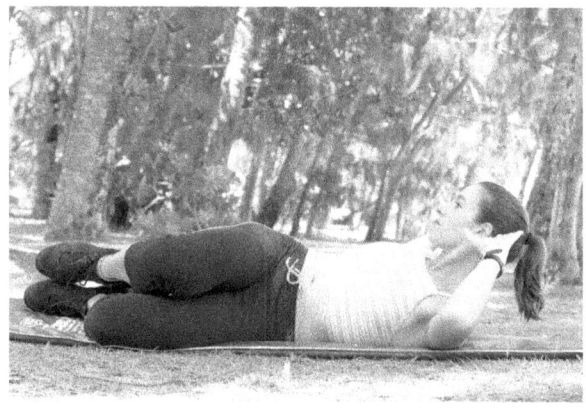

- Lie on your back with one leg straight out along the floor and the other leg lifted with the knee bent.
- Place your hands at the side of your head with your elbows out, and slowly raise the opposite elbow and shoulder up towards the raised leg.
- Complete your reps and swap sides.

REVERSE CURL

Variation is important when working your abdominals, and the reverse curl assists with this variation by working the stomach from the lower part up.

- Lie on your back with palms face down and your arms out to the sides.
- Keeping your head and shoulders on the floor throughout the exercise, lift your legs straight up in the air and back, (no further than your head)
- Now, breathing in contract those abs and bring your pelvis, with your legs, back towards your rib cage in a very slow, controlled movement.
- Hold this position for 2 seconds then lower your legs to the floor (slowly) remembering to breathe out as you go.

OBLIQUE BRIDGE

The oblique bridge is one I prescribe for most of my clients. It can be tough for some, but once mastered, a wonderful exercise for your abdominals.

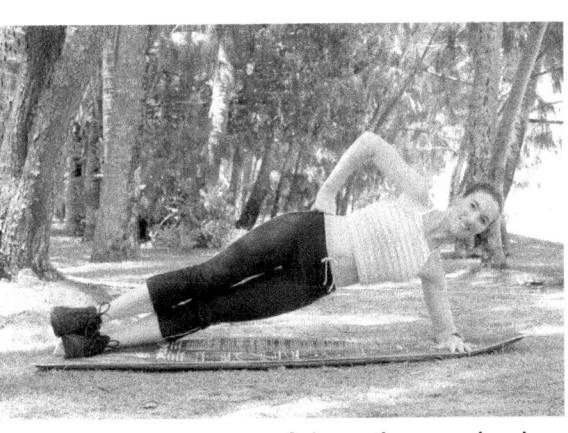

- Place your elbow directly beneath your shoulder to form a solid support.
- With your other arm lying comfortably along your body, place one leg on top of the other and raise yourself up, maintaining a nice straight line from your head to your toes.
- Using your obliques, maintain the position as long you can before lowering to the floor. Repeat each side until required reps are completed.

BRIDGING

THE PRONE BRIDGE

The prone bridge is great for toning up those abs, easy to perfect and no movement required.

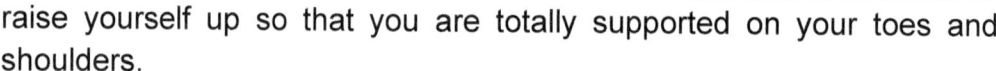

- Lie face down on the floor, on your toes with your elbows directly below your shoulders.
- Maintaining a nice straight line from your feet right through to your shoulders, raise yourself up so that you are totally supported on your toes and shoulders.
- Contracting those abs, hold the position as long as you can before lowering to the starting position.

THE SUPINE BRIDGE

The supine bridge is excellent work for the hamstrings and bum.

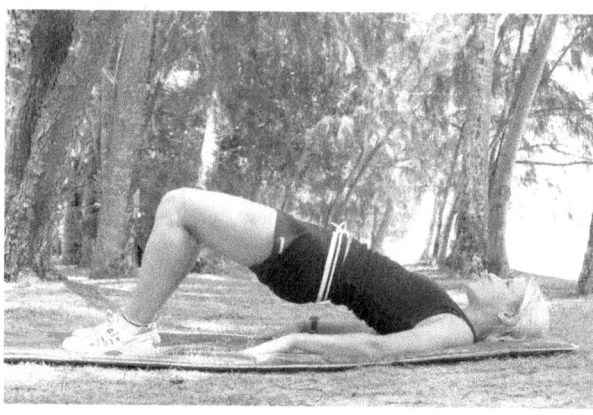

- Lie on your back with the whole length of your spine making contact with the floor.
- Place your hands flat on the floor alongside your hips with your knees bent to 90 degrees.
- Pushing with your feet, lift your bum off the floor as high as you can and hold for 3 seconds, then lower your pelvis without touching the floor and repeat.

SUPINE BRIDGE (VARIATION)

- To increase the intensity, perform exercise with feet up on a bench or a chair with it's back supported against the wall for stability. Alternately, a fitball may be used quite effectively.

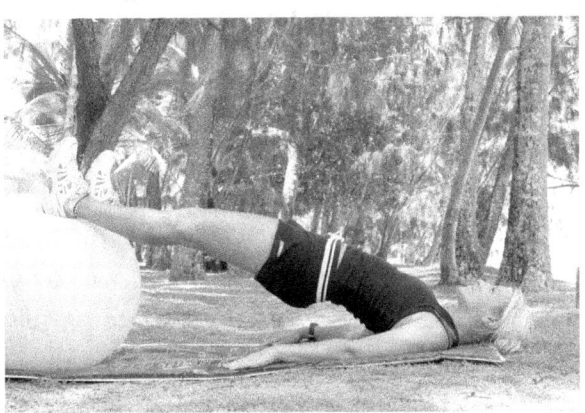

DORSAL RAISE

A pilates based exercise, great for your lower back and the muscles in the lumbar region.

- Lie face down (prone) on the floor with your arms stretched out to the front and and your legs straight out behind you, making sure you're neck is nice and relaxed.

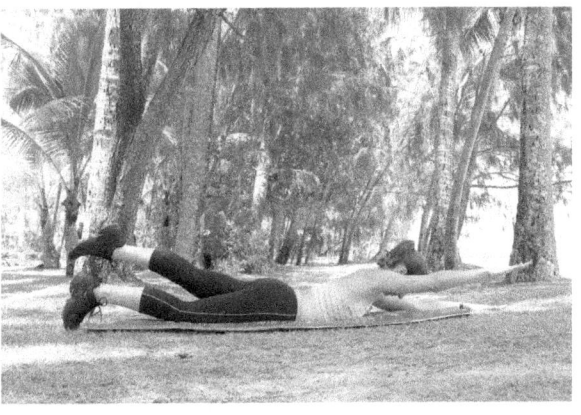

- Raise one leg and one arm together, keeping them straight and breathing out as you go.

- Hold the position for 2 seconds before lowering them slowly back to the starting position, breathing out as you do so.

- Complete alternate reps (one each side until reps are completed)

TORSO LIFTS (STANDING WITH RESISTANCE TUBE)

This exercise will wake up your spinal erectors, hamstrings and gluts (bum)

- Stand with your feet hip-width apart, knees slightly bent and your back straight.
- Place the resistance tube under your feet.
- Now, keeping your arms down by your sides, bend forward from the hip, bringing the torso down until parallel with the floor.
- Breathing out, return to the starting position and repeat the required number of reps.

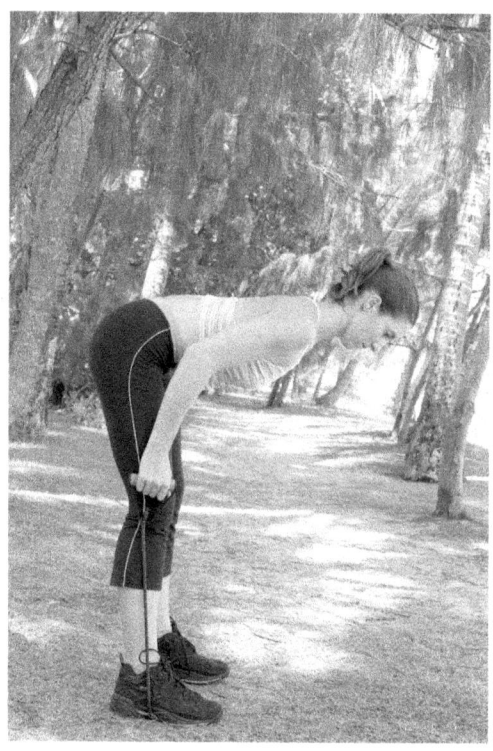

STRETCHING

Exercise involves muscle contraction, causing them to tighten and shorten in length. It is most important to stretch our muscles back to their original length immediately after exercising whilst they are still warm.

Stretching is a habit you must get yourself into. Without it you leave yourself open to injury, reduced flexibility, soreness and stiffness. After every session spend 10 minutes minimum on a full body stretching routine.

FULL BODY STRETCHING SEQUENCE

After a session grab your mat or towel, spread it out on the floor, lay down on your back and stretch out nice and long, oh! what a feeling. Now we will follow the routine below in sequence.

SPINAL ROTATION

Keeping your shoulder blades flat on the floor with your arms stretched out to the sides, bend your legs to 90 degrees. Allow your knees to drop to the floor together, without forcing them and making sure to keep your shoulder blades on the deck. Hold the stretch for 30 seconds minimum before repeating over the other 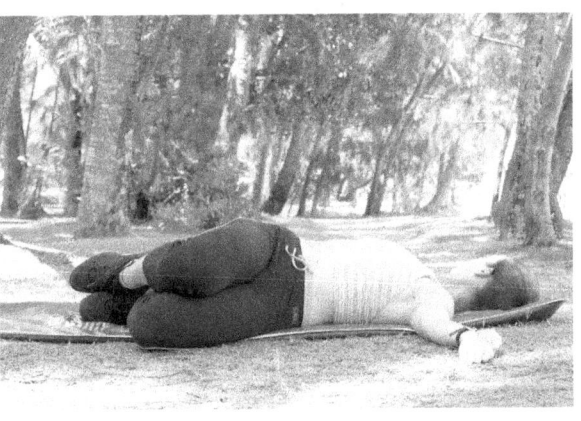 side. Well done, now return to your favourite position(flat on your back) stretch out, relax and prepare for your next stretch.

GLUTEAL STRETCH

Now, keeping one foot on the floor, bend the knee of that leg. Cross the other leg over the first leg so that your ankle is resting above the knee. Reach through and lock your hands around the thigh of your first leg, smoothly pulling back toward you. You will feel a wonderful stretch in your buttocks and outer thigh. Excellent, now

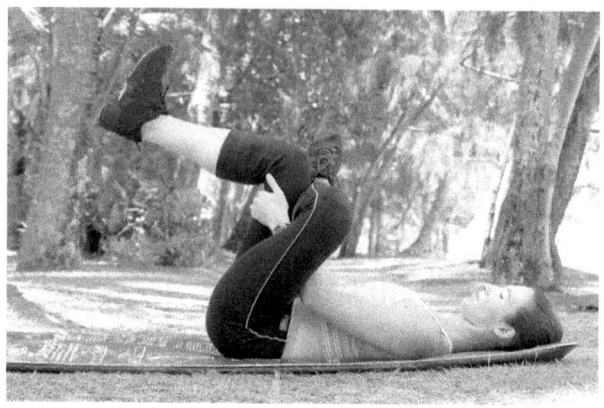

hold that stretch for a minimum of 30 seconds and repeat with the other leg.

QUADRICEP STRETCH

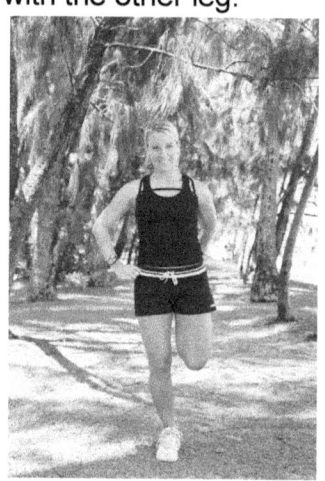

This stretch can be performed either lying or standing. It is important to keep the knees together while performing this stretch. Holding the front of your foot, bring one leg up behind you (actually pulling the heel into your buttock) Hold for a minimum of 30 seconds as you feel the stretch in your hip and thigh.

OUTER THIGH STRETCH

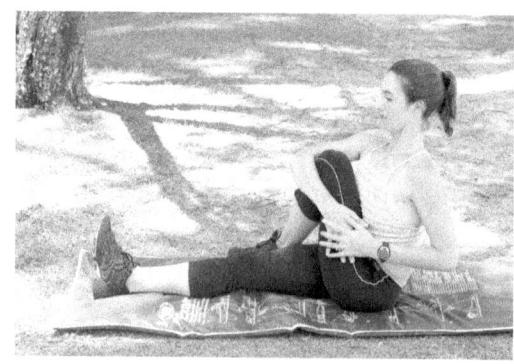

In a sitting position with your legs straight out in front of you, bring one leg up and cross it over the other leg. Supporting yourself with one arm, use the other arm to ease your knee across your body. You will feel the stretch through your outer thigh. Hold the stretch for 30 seconds and repeat with the other leg.

INNER THIGH STRETCH

In a sitting position with your back straight, bring your heels together. Now, holding your ankles, pull your feet in towards you holding the stretch for 30 seconds. You will feel the stretch at your inner thighs as you let your knees drop toward the floor. To intensify this stretch, bring your body gently forward from the hips as you place your elbows on your knees.

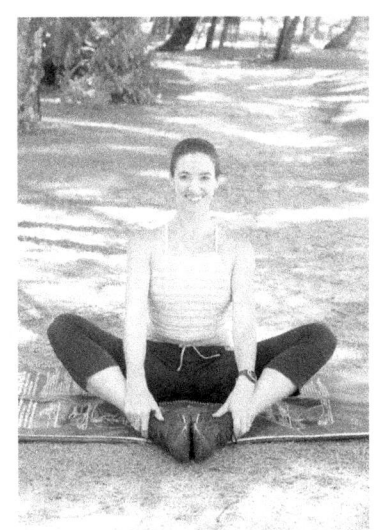

HAMSTRINGS STRETCH

In a sitting position with your legs straight and together, slowly and gently bend forward from the waist with fingers outstretched until you can feel the stretch in your hamstrings. Hold for 30 seconds. If your flexibility is insufficient in the early stages you can assist yourself by folding a towel lengthways, looping it over your feet and holding both ends, gently ease yourself forward.

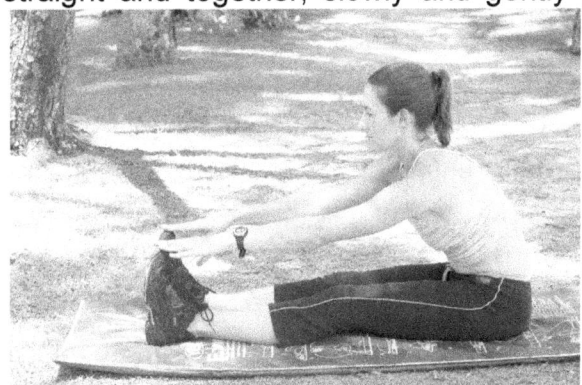

HAMSTRINGS STRETCH (LYING)

Lie on your back with one leg bent to 90 degrees. Bring your other leg straight up toward you and grasp with both hands below the knee. Gently pull the leg toward you until you feel the stretch and hold for 30 seconds minimum.

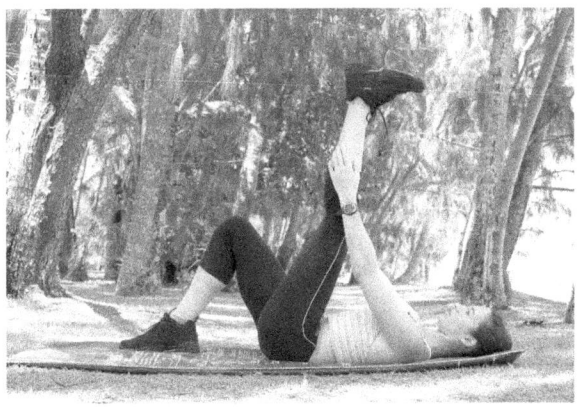

HAMSTRING STRETCH (STANDING)

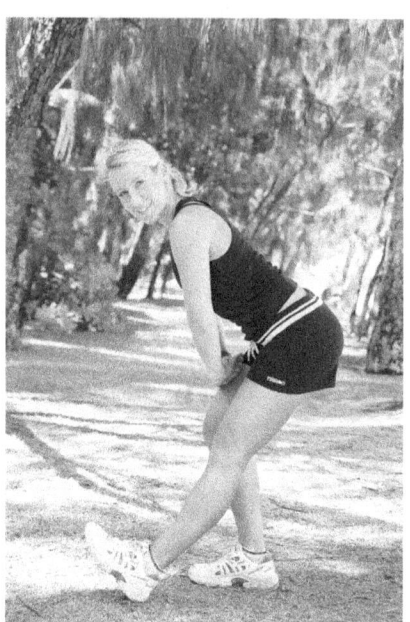

With your hands on your thighs, place one heel in front of you. Bending your other knee slowly bend forward from your hips. You will feel the stretch at the back of your upper leg (hamstring) primarily, with some at the back of the knee and in the calf. Hold the stretch for your minimum 20 seconds, then to intensify the stretch slowly lean a bit further into the stretch, hold for another 20 seconds and repeat for the other leg.

CALF STRETCH

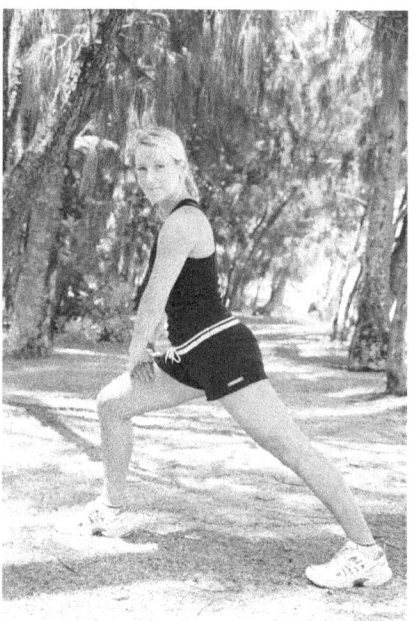

Basically your calf muscle consists of your main muscle, (gastrocnemius) and the lesser (soleus) which is lower and runs underneath. Here are two stretches, one for each respectively.

Standing with your feet together, take a good step back with one leg keeping the foot flat on the deck, with the other leg slightly bent at the knee.

Your upper body weight is taken on the front leg while your feet are facing forward and your back is straight with both heels on the floor.

Intensity can be increased by taking your back leg further back and pushing into the heel. Hold all positions for your 20 seconds minimum and repeat with the other leg.

CALF STRETCH (LOWER)

As with calf stretch above except that the back leg is bent at the knee with the step back being of a shorter distance. The stretch will be felt deep in the lower part of the leg.

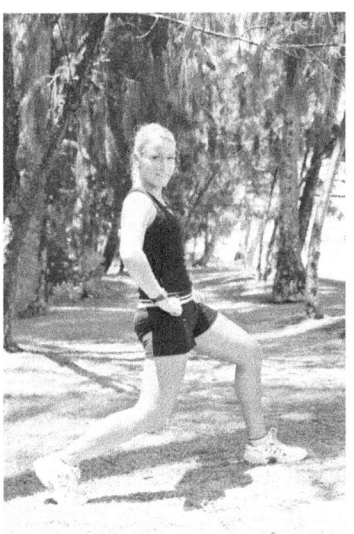

CHEST STRETCH

Sitting with your legs slightly bent and feet hip-width apart, contract those abdominals (pull them in) while relaxing your neck and shoulders.

With your arms straight, interlock your hands behind your back, keeping your back nice and straight.

Now lift your arms up behind you until you feel the stretch across your chest, and hold for at least 20 seconds.

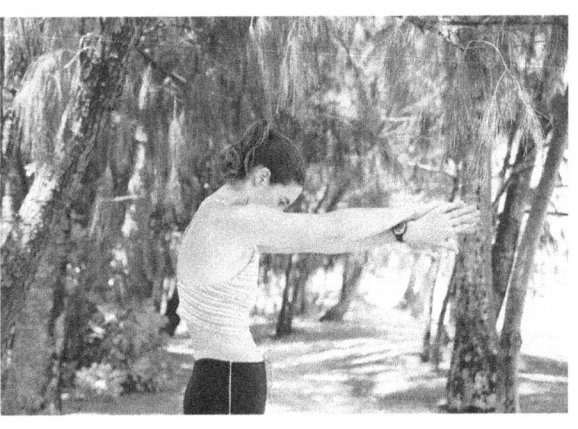

UPPER BACK STRETCH

Standing with your legs slightly bent and feet hip-width apart, tighten those tummy muscles.

Interlocking your fingers together, straighten your arms out in front of you.

Keeping your body upright with a firm lower back, push your hands away from you as you feel the stretch across your upper back and back of your shoulders.

Hold stretch for a minimum of 20 seconds.

TRICEP STRETCH

Standing or seated.

Lifting one arm, place the hand over your back reaching down your spine with fingers pointed downwards.

With your other hand grasp your elbow and gently pull back intensifying the stretch.

Hold for 20 seconds and repeat with other arm.

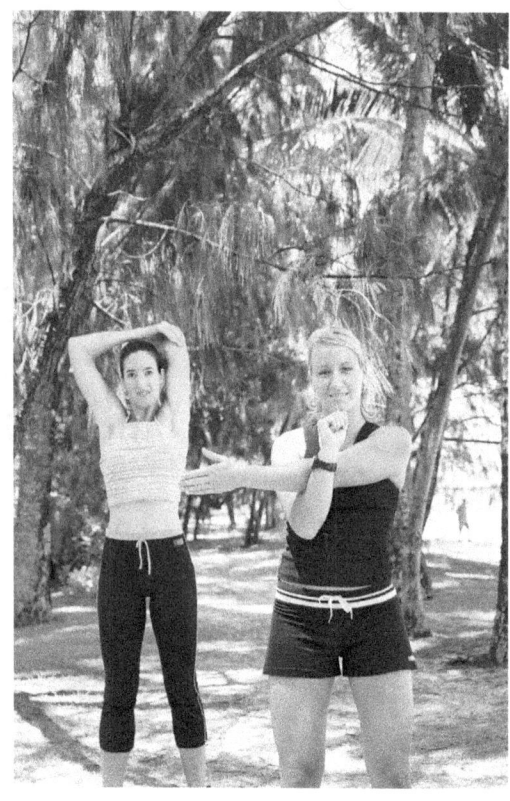

WEEK NO.1   INTENSITY LEVEL: LOW

Day	Resistance Exercise	Page	Reps	Sets	Cardio
Mon	Push up (BOX)	34	Max	1	1/2hr Medium paced walk
	Dorsal raise	55	15	1	Morning and evening
	Step – up	48	15	1	
	Wide squat	48	Max	1	
	Prone bridge	54	15	1	
	Supine bridge	55	15	1	
	Fit ball crunches	52	Max	1	
	Oblique bridge	53	Max	1	
Tues	No resistance work today				As for Monday
Wed	Chest press (TUBE)	33	15	1	35min Medium paced walk
	Seated row (TUBE)	42	15	1	Morning and evening
	Squat (TUBE)	51	15	1	
	Lunge (TUBE)	47	15	1	
	Side leg lifts (TUBE)	49	15	1	
	Prone bridge	54	15	1	
	Supine bridge	55	15	1	
	Fit ball crunches	52	Max	1	
Thur	Bent over raise (TUBE)	35	15	1	35min Medium paced walk
	Upright row (TUBE)	41	15	1	Morning and evening
	Torso lifts (TUBE)	56	15	1	
	Tricep extension (TUBE)	37	15	1	
	Lateral raise (TUBE)	40	15	1	
	Side Bends (TUBE)	52	15	1	
	Oblique crunch	52	Max	1	
	Fit ball crunches	52	Max	1	
Fri	No resistance work today				
Sat	Shoulder press (TUBE)	38	15	1	40min Medium paced walk
	Pec–fly (TUBE)	36	15	1	Morning and evening
	One arm row (TUBE)	43	15	1	
	Bi–cep curl (TUBE)	44	15	1	
	Step and squat	48	Max	1	
	Inner thigh press (TUBE)	49	15	1	
	Power lunge	47	15	1	
	Fit ball crunches	52	Max	1	Sunday rest

WEEK NO.2   INTENSITY LEVEL: LOW

Day	Resistance Exercise	Page	Reps	Sets	Cardio
Mon	Chest press (D-Bells)	33	15	1	45min Medium paced walk
	Pec–fly (TUBE)	36	15	1	Morning & evening or 20min
	Upright row (D-Bells)	41	15	1	Medium paced bike ride(flat)
	Shoulder press (D-Bells)	38	15	1	2 sessions
	Lateral raise (D-Bells)	40	15	1	
	Side bends (TUBE)	52	15	1	
	Oblique crunch	52	Max	1	
	Fit ball crunch	52	Max	2	
Tues	Side lunge	50	15	1	45min Medium paced walk
	Wide squat	48	15	1	Morning & evening or 20min
	Step and squat	48	15	1	Medium paced bike ride(flat)
	Inner thigh press	49	15	1	
	Prone bridge	54	15	1	
	Supine bridge	55	15	1	
	Dorsal raise	55	15	1	
	Fit ball crunches	52	Max	2	
Wed	Upright row (TUBE)	41	15	1	45min Medium paced walk or
	Bent over raise (TUBE)	35	15	1	20min Medium paced bike ride
	Seated row (TUBE)	42	15	1	Or aerobic or aqua class
	Alternate D-Bells curls	45	15	1	2 sessions
	One arm row (D-Bells)	43	15	1	
	Oblique bridge	54	10	1	
	Reverse curl	53	Max	1	
	Fit ball crunches	52	Max	2	
Thur	No resistance work today				
Fri	Chest press (TUBE)	33	15	1	
	Push up	34	Max	1	As for Wednesday
	Pec–fly (TUBE)	36	15	1	
	Tricep kickback	37	15	1	
	Side bends (TUBE)	52	15	1	
	Torso lifts (TUBE)	56	15	1	
	Reverse curl	53	Max	1	
	Fit ball crunches	52	Max	2	
Sat	Squat (TUBE)	51	15	1	
	Lunge (TUBE)	47	15	1	Medium intensity
	Step and squat	48	15	1	2 sessions
	Side leg lifts	49	15	1	
	Side bends (TUBE)	52	15	1	
	Oblique crunch	52	Max	1	
	Dorsal raise	55	Max	1	
	Fit ball crunches	52	Max	2	Sunday rest

WEEK NO.3　INTENSITY LEVEL: LOW

Day	Resistance Exercise	Page	Reps	Sets	Cardio
Mon	Chest press (D-Bells)	33	20	1	Either: 40min walk/run
	Push ups	34	Max	1	25min bike
	Pec–fly	36	20	1	25min swim
	Tricep extension (TUBE)	37	20	1	1 hr class, aerobic/aqua
	Shoulder press (D-Bells)	38	20	1	2 sessions
	Lateral raise (D-Bells)	40	20	1	
	Reverse curls	53	Max	2	
	Fit ball crunches	52	Max	2	
Tues	Squat (TUBE)	51	20	1	As for Monday
	Step and squat	48	20	1	
	Side lunge	50	20	1	
	Inner thigh press	49	20	1	
	Side leg lifts	49	20	1	
	Oblique bridge	53	15	1	
	Supine bridge	55	15	1	
	Fit ball crunches	52	Max	2	
Wed	No resistance work today		Max	1	As for Monday
Thur	Seated row (TUBE)	42	20	1	As for Monday
	Upright row (D-Bells)	41	20	1	
	Bent over raise (TUBE)	35	20	1	
	Bi–cep curl (D-Bells)	35	20	1	
	Hammer curl (TUBE)	45	20	1	
	Oblique crunch	52	Max	2	
	Side bends (TUBE)	52	20	1	
	Fit ball crunches	52	Max	2	
Fri	Knee raise	50	20	1	As for Monday
	Wide squat	48	20	1	
	Power lunge	47	20	1	
	Side lunge	50	20	1	
	Reverse curl	53	Max	2	
	Supine bridge (F-Ball)	55	Max	2	
	Oblique bridge	54	Max	2	
	Fit ball crunches	52	Max	2	
Sat	No resistance work today				Cardio optional
					WEEKEND OFF

WEEK NO.4   INTENSITY LEVEL: LOW

Day	Resistance Exercise	Page	Reps	Sets	Cardio
Mon	Push ups	34	Max	1	Either: 45min walk/run
	Chest press (TUBE)	33	25	1	20min run
	Pec–fly	36	25	1	30min bike
	Tricep kickback (D-Bells)	37	25	1	30min swim
	Tricep extension (TUBE)	37	25	1	1 hr class, aerobic/aqua
	Oblique bridge	54	Max	2	2 sessions
	Side bends (TUBE)	52	25	1	
	Fit ball crunches	52	Max	2	
Tues	Squat (TUBE)	51	25	1	As for Monday
	Wide squat	48	25	1	
	Step and squat	48	25	1	
	Knee raise	50	25	1	
	Side lunge	50	25	1	
	Dorsal raise	55	25	1	
	Oblique bridge	53	15	1	
	Fit ball crunches	52	Max	2	
Wed	Bent over raise (TUBE)	35	25	1	As for Monday
	Upright row (TUBE)	41	25	1	
	Seated row (TUBE)	42	25	1	
	One arm row (TUBE)	43	25	1	
	Bi–cep curl (TUBE)	44	25	1	
	Oblique crunch	52	Max	2	
	Oblique bridge	54	Max	2	
	Side Bends	52	25	1	
Thur	No resistance work today				As for Monday
Fri	Chest press (D-Bells)	33	25	1	As for Monday
	Push ups	34	Max	1	
	Pec–fly	36	25	1	
	Tricep extension (TUBE)	37	25	1	
	Shoulder press (TUBE)	38	25	1	
	Lateral raise (D-Bells)	40	25	1	
	Reverse curls	53	Max	2	
	Fit ball crunches	52	Max	2	
Sat	Squat (TUBE)	51	25	1	As for Monday
	Lunge (TUBE)	47	25	1	
	Side leg lifts	49	25	1	
	Inner thigh press	49	25	1	
	Reverse curl	53	Max	2	
	Oblique crunch	52	Max	2	
	Supine bridge (F-Ball)	55	Max	2	
	Fit ball crunches	52	Max	2	Sunday rest

WEEK NO.5   INTENSITY LEVEL: MEDIUM

Day	Resistance Exercise	Page	Reps	Sets	Cardio
Mon	Seated row (TUBE)	42	15	2	Choice of:50min walk/run
	Bent over raise (TUBE)	35	15	2	20min run
	Upright row (D-Bells)	41	15	2	30min bike
	One arm row (D-Bells)	43	15	2	30min swim
	Bi–cep curl (TUBE)	44	15	2	1 hr class/aerobic/aqua
	Hammer curls (D-Bells)	45	15	2	2 sessions
	Oblique crunches	52	Max	2	
	Fit ball crunches	52	Max	2	
Tues	Squat (TUBE)	51	15	2	As for Monday
	Step and squat	48	15	2	
	Side lunge	50	15	2	
	Inner thigh press	49	15	2	
	Side leg lifts	49	15	2	
	Oblique bridge	53	15	2	
	Supine bridge	55	15	2	
	Fit ball crunches	52	Max	2	
	Dorsal raise	55	15	1	
Wed	No resistance work today				As for Monday
Thur	Chest press (D-Bells)	33	15	2	
	Push ups	34	Max	2	
	Pec-fly	36	15	2	
	Shoulder press (D-Bells)	38	15	2	
	Lateral raise (D-Bells)	40	15	2	
	Reverse curls	53	15	2	
	Side Bends	52	15	2	
	Fit ball crunches	52	Max	2	
Fri	Knee raise	50	15	2	
	Power lunge	47	15	2	
	Wide squat	48	15	2	
	Side lunge	50	15	2	
	Oblique crunches	52	Max	2	
	Oblique bridge	53	15	2	
	Dorsal raise	55	15	2	
	Fit ball crunches	52	15	2	
Sat	No resistance work today				Cardio optional
					WEEKEND OFF

WEEK NO.6   INTENSITY LEVEL: MEDIUM

Day	Resistance Exercise	Page	Reps	Sets	Cardio
Mon	Bent over raise (TUBE)	35	15	2	Choice of:50min walk/run
	Upright row (TUBE)	41	15	2	20min run
	Seated row (TUBE)	42	15	2	30min bike
	One-arm row (TUBE)	43	15	2	30min swim
	Hammer curls (TUBE)	45	15	2	1 hr class aerobic/aqua
	Torso lifts	56	15	2	2 sessions
	Prone bridge	54	15	2	
	Fit ball crunches	52	Max	3	
Tues	Squat (TUBE)	51	15	2	As for Monday
	Knee raise	50	15	2	
	Wide squat	48	15	2	
	Side lunge	50	15	2	
	Side bends (TUBE)	52	15	2	
	Oblique crunches	52	Max	2	
	Dorsal raise	55	15	1	
	Fit ball crunches	52	Max	2	
Wed	Chest press (TUBE)	33	15	2	As for Monday
	Pec-fly (TUBE)	36	15	2	
	Push-ups	34	15	2	
	Tricep extension (TUBE)	37	15	2	
	Tricep kickback (D-Bells)	37	15	2	
	Prone bridge	54	15	2	
	Oblique crunches	52	Max	3	
Thur	No resistance work today				As for Monday
Fri	Upright row (D-Bells)	41	15	2	As for Monday
	Bent over raise (D-Bells)	35	15	2	
	Seated row (TUBE)	42	15	2	
	One-arm row (D-Bells)	43	15	2	
	Bi–cep curls (TUBE)	44	15	2	
	Oblique bridge	54	15	2	
	Fit ball crunches	52	Max	2	
Sat	Squat (TUBE)	51	15	2	As for Monday
	Step and squat	48	15	2	
	Side lunge	50	15	2	
	Side leg lifts	49	15	2	
	Inner thigh press	49	15	2	
	Reverse curls	53	15	2	
	Dorsal raise	55	15	2	
	Fit ball crunches	52	Max	3	Sunday rest

WEEK NO.7   INTENSITY LEVEL: MEDIUM

Day	Resistance Exercise	Page	Reps	Sets	Cardio
Mon	Chest press (D-Bells)	33	20	2	Choice of:50min walk/run
	Push-ups	34	Max	2	25min run
	Pec–fly (TUBE)	36	20	2	35min bike
	Shoulder press (TUBE)	38	20	2	35min swim
	Lateral raise (TUBE)	40	20	2	1 hr class aqua/pilates
	Tricep kickback (D-Bells)	37	20	2	
	Reverse curls	53	20	2	
	Fit ball crunch	52	Max	3	
Tues	Step and squat	48	20	2	As for Monday
	Squat (TUBE)	51	20	2	
	Side lunge	50	20	2	
	Inner thigh press	49	20	2	
	Side leg lifts	49	20	2	
	Oblique bridge	53	20	2	
	Dorsal raise	55	20	2	
	Oblique crunches	52	Max	3	
Wed	No resistance work today				As for Monday
Thur	Seated row (TUBE)	42	20	2	As for Monday
	Upright row (D-Bells)	41	20	2	
	Bent over raise (TUBE)	35	20	2	
	One arm row (TUBE)	43	20	2	
	Bi–cep curl (D-Bells)	44	20	2	
	Hammer curls (D-Bells)	45	20	2	
	Supine bridge	55	20	2	
	Fit ball crunches	52	Max	3	
Fri	Power lunge	47	20	2	As for Monday
	Wide squat	48	20	2	
	Step and squat	48	20	2	
	Side lunge	50	20	2	
	Side bends	52	20	2	
	Reverse curls	53	20	2	
	Fit ball crunches	52	Max	2	
Sat	No resistance work today				Cardio optional
					WEEK END OFF

WEEK NO.8   INTENSITY LEVEL: MEDIUM

Day	Resistance Exercise	Page	Reps	Sets	Cardio
Mon	Chest press (D-Bells)	33	25	2	Choice of:50min walk/run
	Push-ups	34	Max	2	25min run
	Pec–fly (TUBE)	36	25	2	35min bike
	Tricep extension (TUBE)	37	25	2	35min swim
	Tricep kickback	37	25	2	1 hr class aqua/aerobic
	Reverse curl	53	25	2	2 sessions
	Oblique bridge	54	25	2	
	Fit ball crunches	52	Max	2	
Tues	Squat (TUBE)	51	25	2	As for Monday
	Step and squat	48	25	2	
	Side lunge	50	25	2	
	Inner thigh press	49	25	2	
	Side leg lifts	49	25	2	
	Supine bridge	55	25	2	
	Prone bridge	54	25	2	
	Oblique crunches	52	Max	3	
Wed	Upright row (TUBE)	41	25	2	As for Monday
	Seated row (TUBE)	42	25	2	
	Bent over raise (TUBE)	35	25	2	
	One arm row	43	25	2	
	Bi–cep curl (D-Bells)	44	25	2	
	Side-bends	52	25	2	
	Torso lifts	56	25	2	
	Dorsal raise	55	25	2	
Thur	No resistance work today				As for Monday
Fri	Chest press (TUBE)	33	25	2	As for Monday
	Pec–fly (TUBE)	36	25	2	
	Push-ups	34	Max	2	
	Shoulder press (D-Bells)	38	25	2	
	Lateral raise (TUBE)	40	25	2	
	Reverse curls	53	25	2	
	Oblique bridge	54	25	2	
	Fit ball crunches	52	Max	3	
Sat	Squat (TUBE)	51	25	2	As for Monday
	Wide-squat	48	25	2	
	Knee raise	50	25	2	
	Side lunge	50	25	2	
	Side bends	52	25	2	
	Dorsal raise	55	25	2	
	Fit ball crunches	52	Max	2	
	Oblique crunches	54	Max	2	WEEK END OFF

WEEK NO.9   INTENSITY LEVEL: HIGH

Day	Resistance Exercise	Page	Reps	Sets	Cardio
Mon	Seated row (TUBE)	42	15	3	Choice of:50min brisk walk
	Upright row (D-Bells)	41	15	3	30min run
	One arm row (D-Bells)	43	15	3	40min bike
	Bent over raise (TUBE)	35	15	3	40min swim
	Hammer curls (D-Bells)	45	15	3	1 hr class
	Bi–cep curl (D-Bells Alt)	45	15	3	2 sessions
	Oblique bridge	54	15	3	
	Oblique crunch	52	Max	3	
Tues	Squat (TUBE)	51	15	3	As for Monday
	Side lunge	50	15	3	
	Step and squat	48	15	3	
	Inner thigh press	49	15	3	
	Side leg lifts	49	15	3	
	Reverse curls	53	15	3	
	Prone bridge	54	15	3	
	Fit ball crunches	52	Max	3	
Wed	No resistance work today				As for Monday
Thur	Chest press (D-Bells)	33	15	3	As for Monday
	Push-ups	34	Max	3	
	Peck-fly(TUBE)	36	15	3	
	Tricep extension (TUBE)	37	15	3	
	Tricep kickback (D-Bells)	37	15	3	
	Supine bridge	55	15	3	
	Oblique bridge	54	15	3	
	Fit ball crunches	52	Max	3	
Fri	Squat (TUBE)	51	15	3	As for Monday
	Knee raise	50	15	3	
	Side lunge	50	15	3	
	Wide squat	48	15	3	
	Dorsal raise	55	15	3	
	Torso lifts	56	15	3	
	Reverse curls	53	15	3	
	Fit ball crunches	52	Max	3	
Sat	No resistance work today				Cardio optional
					WEEK END OFF

WEEK NO.10   INTENSITY LEVEL: HIGH

Day	Resistance Exercise	Page	Reps	Sets	Cardio
3	Seated row (TUBE)	42	15	3	Choice of:50min brisk walk
	Upright row (TUBE)	41	15	3	30min run
	Bent over raise (TUBE)	35	15	3	40min bike
	One arm row (D-Bells)	43	15	3	40min swim
	Bi–cep curl (TUBE)	44	15	3	1 hr class
	Alternate Bi-cep curls (D-Bells)	45	15	3	2 sessions
	Reverse curls	53	15	3	
	Fit ball crunches	52	15	3	
	Oblique crunch	52	Max	3	
Tues	Squat (TUBE)	51	15	3	As for Monday
	Single leg squat	46	10	3	
	Side lunge	50	15	3	
	Inner thigh press	49	15	3	
	Side leg lifts	49	15	3	
	Oblique bridge	54	15	3	
	Prone bridge	54	15	3	
	Fit ball crunches	52	15	3	
Wed	Chest press (TUBE)	33	15	3	As for Monday
	Push-ups	34	Max	3	
	Peck-fly(TUBE)	36	15	3	
	Shoulder press (TUBE)	38	15	3	
	Lateral raise	40	15	3	
	Tricep extension (TUBE)	37	15	3	
	Oblique crunches	52	Max	3	
	Reverse curls	53	15	3	
Thur	No resistance work today				As for Monday
Fri	Single leg squats	46	10	3	
	Squat (TUBE)	51	15	3	
	Knee raise	50	15	3	
	Side lunge	50	15	3	
	Wide squat	48	15	3	
	Torso lifts	56	15	3	
	Fit ball crunches	52	Max	3	
	Oblique bridge	54	15	3	
Sat	Upright row (TUBE)	41	15	3	
	Bent over raise (TUBE)	35	15	3	
	Alternate Bi-cep curls (D-Bells)	45	15	3	
	Hammer curls (TUBE)	45	15	3	
	Reverse curls (TUBE)	53	15	3	
	Fit ball crunches	52	Max	3	SUNDAY REST

WEEK NO.11   INTENSITY LEVEL: HIGH

Day	Resistance Exercise	Page	Reps	Sets	Cardio
Mon	Chest press (D-Bells)	33	20	3	Choice of:50min brisk walk
	Push-ups	34	Max	3	30min run
	Pec–fly (TUBE)	36	20	3	40min bike
	Tricep extension (TUBE)	37	20	3	40min swim
	Tricep kickback (D-Bells)	37	20	3	1 hr class
	Prone bridge	54	20	3	2 sessions
	Oblique bridge	54	20	3	
	Fit ball crunch	52	Max	3	
Tues	Squat (TUBE)	51	20	3	As for Monday
	Single leg squat	46	12	3	
	Inner thigh press	49	20	3	
	Side leg lifts	49	20	3	
	Step and squat	48	20	3	
	Reverse curls	53	20	3	
	Oblique crunches	52	20	3	
	Fit ball crunches	52	Max	3	
Wed	No resistance work today				As for Monday
Thur	Seated row (TUBE)	42	20	3	As for Monday
	Upright row (TUBE)	41	20	3	
	Bent over raise (TUBE)	35	20	3	
	One arm row (D-Bells)	43	20	3	
	Bi–cep curls (D-Bells)	44	20	3	
	Supine bridge	55	20	3	
	Torso lifts	56	20	3	
	Fit ball crunches	52	Max	3	
Fri	Squat (TUBE)	51	20	3	As for Monday
	Side lunge	50	20	3	
	Step and squat	48	20	3	
	Side bends	52	20	3	
	Reverse curls	53	Max	3	
	Oblique bridge	54	20	3	
	Fit ball crunches	52	Max	3	
	Dorsal raise	55	20	3	
Sat	No resistance work today				Cardio optional
					WEEK END OFF

WEEK NO.12　INTENSITY LEVEL: HIGH

Day	Resistance Exercise	Page	Reps	Sets	Cardio
Mon	Chest press (D-Bells)	33	25	3	Choice of:1 hr brisk walk
	Pec–fly (TUBE)	36	25	3	35min run
	Push-ups	34	Max	3	45min bike
	Shoulder press (D-Bells)	38	25	3	45min swim
	Lateral raise (D-Bells)	40	25	3	1 hr class
	Oblique bridge	54	25	3	2 sessions
	Supine bridge	54	25	3	
	Fit ball crunches	52	Max	3	
Tues	Squat (TUBE)	51	25	3	As for Monday
	Single leg squat	46	15	3	
	Side lunge	50	25	3	
	Power lunge	47	25	3	
	Inner thigh press	49	25	3	
	Side leg lifts	49	25	3	
	Reverse curls	53	25	3	
	Fit ball crunches	52	Max	3	
Wed	Seated row (TUBE)	42	25	3	As for Monday
	Upright row (D-Bells)	41	25	3	
	One arm row (D-Bells)	43	25	3	
	Alternate Bi-cep curls (D-Bells)	45	25	3	
	Bi–cep curls (D-Bells)	44	25	3	
	Oblique crunches	52	Max	3	
	Torso lifts	56	25	3	
	Prone bridge	54	25	3	
Thur	No resistance work today				As for Monday
Fri	Squat (TUBE)	51	25	3	As for Monday
	Step and squat	48	25	3	
	Side lunge	50	25	3	
	Knee raise	50	25	3	
	Torso lifts	56	25	3	
	Side bends	52	25	3	
	Reverse curls	53	25	3	
	Fit ball crunches	52	Max	3	
Sat	Chest press (D-Bells)	33	25	3	As for Monday
	Push-ups	34	Max	3	
	Pec–fly	36	25	3	
	Oblique bridge	54	25	3	
	Tricep extension (TUBE)	37	25	3	
	Tricep kickback	37	25	3	
	Oblique bridge	54	25	3	
	Side bends	52	25	3	
	Reverse curls	53	Max	3	SUNDAY REST

www.ingramcontent.com/pod-product-compliance
Lightning Source LLC
Chambersburg PA
CBHW052007280526
45793CB00005B/878